DIGITAL TRANSFORMATION IN HEALTHCARE

Digital Transformation: Accelerating Organizational Intelligence

Print ISSN: 2811-0552
Online ISSN: 2811-0560

Series Editor: Jay Liebowitz *(Rollins College, USA)*

According to a report released by Veritis in 2021 "the global digital transformation market size is anticipated to reach USD 1009.8 billion by 2025 from USD 469.8 billion in 2020. The demand for digital transformation services is expected to rise at a Compound Annual Growth Rate (CAGR) of around 16.5% over the forecast period from 2021 to 2025. The growing adoption of digital technologies, including Artificial Intelligence (AI), cloud computing, big data, the Internet of Things (IoT), and Machine Learning (ML), is driving the growth of the digital transformation market." To be competitive in today's fast-changing marketplace, organizations need to apply the "alphabet" of digital transformation.

The focus of the book series is unique and will cover the various perspectives on organizational digital transformation, namely business & management, technology, legal and ethics, and social aspects.

Published:

Vol. 9   *Digital Transformation in Healthcare*
edited by Jay Liebowitz

Vol. 8   *Achieving Digital Transformation through Analytics and AI*
edited by Jay Liebowitz

Vol. 7   *Digital Transformation and Society*
edited by Jay Liebowitz

Vol. 6   *Strategic Risk, Intelligence and Digital Transformation*
by Eduardo Rodriguez

Vol. 5   *Digital Transformation for Entrepreneurship*
edited by Susanne Durst and Aive Pevkur

Vol. 4   *Digital Strategies and Organizational Transformation*
edited by G Reza Djavanshir

Vol. 3   *Doing Well and Doing Good: Human-Centered Digital Transformation Leadership*
by Cheryl Flink, Liora Gross and William Pasmore

Vol. 2   *Digital Transformation Demystified*
by Frank Granito

More information on this series can be found at https://www.worldscientific.com/series/dtaoi

Digital Transformation
Accelerating Organizational Intelligence
– Volume 9

DIGITAL TRANSFORMATION IN HEALTHCARE

Edited by

Jay Liebowitz
Rollins College, USA

World Scientific

NEW JERSEY · LONDON · SINGAPORE · BEIJING · SHANGHAI · HONG KONG · TAIPEI · CHENNAI · TOKYO

Published by

World Scientific Publishing Co. Pte. Ltd.

5 Toh Tuck Link, Singapore 596224

USA office: 27 Warren Street, Suite 401-402, Hackensack, NJ 07601

UK office: 57 Shelton Street, Covent Garden, London WC2H 9HE

Library of Congress Cataloging-in-Publication Data

Names: Liebowitz, Jay, 1957- editor

Title: Digital transformation in healthcare / edited by Jay Liebowitz, Rollins College, USA.

Description: New Jersey : World Scientific, [2026] | Series: Digital
   transformation : accelerating organizational intelligence, 2811-0552 |
   Includes bibliographical references and index.

Identifiers: LCCN 2025012320 | ISBN 9789819813490 hardcover |
   ISBN 9789819813506 ebook for institutions | ISBN 9789819813513 ebook for individuals

Subjects: LCSH: Medical informatics--Technological innovations |
   Artificial intelligence--Medical applications

Classification: LCC R858 .D544 2025

LC record available at https://lccn.loc.gov/2025012320

British Library Cataloguing-in-Publication Data

A catalogue record for this book is available from the British Library.

Copyright © 2026 by World Scientific Publishing Co. Pte. Ltd.

For any available supplementary material, please visit
https://www.worldscientific.com/worldscibooks/10.1142/14323#t=suppl

Desk Editors: Kannan Krishnan/Catherine Domingo Ong/Monali Ghanekar

Typeset by Stallion Press
Email: enquiries@stallionpress.com

To our son, Jason Liebowitz, MD, and our daughter-in-law, Anat Chemerinski, MD, who will continue to face the exciting times ahead in the digital transformation in healthcare.

Foreword: An Industry Perspective by Tom Nesteruk

I was excited when recently asked by my business colleague (and the editor of this book) to participate on a newly created Artificial Intelligence Advisory Board at his college. Being a human resources executive for one of the country's largest not-for-profit healthcare organizations, I have seen and experienced a slow but steady shift during the past five years in how healthcare systems are using and plan to further utilize technology (including AI) – both for patients and team members alike. Having worked in other industries prior to healthcare (aerospace defense, big pharma, and telecommunications), I can certainly attest that the healthcare industry has generally lagged when it comes to utilizing and leveraging modern technology. From hospitals still using pen and paper for patient charts to payrolls being processed off Excel spreadsheets, the industry has fallen behind the times. This idling in digital modernization was never more prevalent than during the COVID-19 pandemic, which brought about unprecedented challenges across the industry.

Working in healthcare during the pandemic, operational inefficiencies became exposed more than ever. While the initial priority was focused on the care and treatment of our patients, it then quickly shifted to human resources and team member wellness. Staffing became the highest priority, due to the shortage of nurses. Physician and nurse burnout also became prevalent and posed many challenges. There was nothing more critical than making sure each one of our hospitals had sufficient resources so that they could care for the communities that we serve.

To achieve this, it was necessary to become more efficient in how we operate and leverage technology to do so. A prime example in my organization was the rapid creation of an employee portal that listed all our hospitals and the available nursing shifts that needed to be covered. For the first time ever, nurses from across the organization could virtually register (via a mobile phone app) and pick up available shifts at any of our various locations. While it may not appear to be that significant of advancement in technology, keep in mind that every shift covered meant that a patient was being treated and not turned away. In addition, our hospitals across the country were utilizing virtual patient care (telehealth) more so than ever before, out of necessity brought on by the pandemic. No longer was it necessary to have to physically be seen by a medical provider. A diagnosis could be determined much quicker and without the long wait times. Both patients and physicians were forced to adjust to this new way of medical care. The medical community, like the rest of the world, recognized that work could still get done and patients treated – albeit on a virtual platform. The pandemic clearly set the stage for healthcare to recognize that the industry needed to digitally transform.

Fast forward to today and most likely you've been in some type of conversation around artificial intelligence. It's unavoidable, especially in healthcare. Hospital CEOs have now prioritized the importance of technology because of AI and how it will change the landscape of patient care. Think about what is occurring right now with our aging population. In 2024, about 4.1 million Americans turned 65, which is a record high. This surge is predicted to continue through 2027 (known as Peak 65) and will have the heaviest impact ever on this country's retirement system. It will totally change the payer–provider mix in healthcare, with significantly more medical reimbursements coming from the government's medicare program versus commercial health insurance (medicare typically provides lower reimbursements due to predetermined rates). Further complicating this scenario is the forecasted physician/nursing shortage. Thus, healthcare CEOs are scrambling to figure out how to integrate AI and other technologies to offset the predicted loss of revenue, staffing challenges, and labor costs. Hospital leadership, whether clinical or non-clinical, must change their way of thinking as it relates to the use of technology and how it can be applied to the patient setting along with team member wellbeing.

As a human resources healthcare executive with an extensive background in HR technology, I, like my fellow colleagues, am always looking for ways to better position my organization. About a year and a half ago,

I led a project that entailed our organization in being one of the first to utilize a component of AI for recruiting in healthcare. Suffice to say, AI technology helped us gain efficiency in our recruitment process, along with providing a strong return on investment. An interesting feature of the technology involves AI constantly searching your candidate database and matching up prior applicants to newly created job requisitions. In the past, this would have taken a tremendous amount of time and manual effort or not happened at all. The implementation of this technology has initiated the onset of a cultural and mindset shift within our organization as it pertains to digital transformation.

This book delves into the digital transformation of healthcare. It is a timely and necessary read that addresses the need for healthcare systems to adapt their strategies around technology to remain competitive and provide the highest levels of patient care. From the demographic and workforce changes caused by an ever-increasing aging population to the probable revisions of healthcare policy by a new incoming administration, healthcare providers will need to be prepared to operate under incredibly challenging times. With this work, the authors have provided invaluable insights and perspectives so that we recognize and can then plan for the impact of the transformed digital landscape in healthcare. I am confident this work will inspire further conversation and exploration in the field.

Tom Nesteruk
Senior Vice President, Human Resources
AdventHealth

Foreword: An Academic Perspective by Jay Spitulnik and Marie Maloney

The digital transformation of healthcare can drive significant change in its delivery. This book delves into the dynamic and evolving world of digital health technology and its impact on healthcare. You will see how technology is changing patient care, enhancing medical research, and empowering individuals to take charge of their health. We hope you see what we see: a future where digital technology delivers higher quality care for every person in the global community.

In the face of aging populations, rising healthcare costs, and increasing disease burdens, healthcare systems worldwide are grappling with significant challenges. To address these universal issues, we require innovative solutions that go beyond traditional healthcare models. We need to rewire how healthcare is delivered. Digital transformation offers a global approach to enhance healthcare access, improve quality, and ensure sustainability. Digital health technologies address the challenges healthcare currently is, and will be, dealing with and create a more resilient and equitable healthcare landscape.

As the world's population ages, demands on global healthcare systems are increasing because more patients need substantial care and management of chronic diseases. At the same time, the need for advanced treatments and increased life expectancies are leading to rising costs. Digital health technologies, including solutions such as electronic health records, telemedicine, remote monitoring, and artificial intelligence (AI) provide us with an opportunity to provide more efficient and effective care delivery.

The landscape of digital health is incredibly diverse, with a wide range of technologies being applied across different countries and regions. From AI-driven diagnostic tools that enhance the accuracy of medical imaging to telemedicine platforms that connect patients in remote areas with specialists in urban centers, digital health innovations are transforming healthcare delivery worldwide. Successful case studies from various parts of the world highlight the transformative potential of these technologies. Estonia's nationwide electronic health record system has streamlined patient care and improved health outcomes leading to a higher quality of life. In Rwanda, drone technology delivers essential medical supplies to remote areas, ensuring timely access to life-saving treatments. These examples underscore the importance of adapting digital health solutions to local contexts to maximize their impact.

Technologies such as AI and machine learning, the Internet of Medical Things (IoMT), and blockchain have the potential to support revolutionary changes to how we manage healthcare, and we've only scratched the surface of how these technologies can transform healthcare:

- AI and machine learning are enhancing diagnostic accuracy and personalizing treatment plans for cancer patients. Analyzing vast amounts of medical data to identify patterns and predict disease outbreaks enables proactive public health interventions. Use of AI in clinical decision support systems allows for the creation of personalized treatment plans based on individual patient data resulting in better outcomes and reduced costs.
- IoMT devices enable continuous health monitoring and early intervention and allow patients to recover at home instead of at the hospital thereby reducing infection risks. Wearable health monitors provide real-time data on patient health allowing for timely treatment and reduced hospital readmissions.
- Blockchain technology ensures secure and transparent data management, fostering trust and collaboration among stakeholders. The decentralized and secure nature of blockchain technology can ensure the confidentiality of patient data and, in turn, support the drive toward interoperability facilitating data sharing across healthcare systems securely.

Government policies and regulations play a crucial role in the adoption and implementation of digital health technologies. Supportive regulatory frameworks are essential to encourage innovation, investment, and safe integration of new technologies into healthcare. Policies that promote interoperability, protect patient privacy, and safeguard the security of patient data, while ensuring equitable access, are vital for the successful digital transformation of healthcare. Government support for the development and deployment of digital health solutions through funding and public–private partnerships is critical and leads to innovation in healthcare delivery and outcomes.

Data is the lifeblood of the digital transformation of healthcare. Currently, much of patient data collected by one provider is not easily accessed by others involved in the patient's care. Data sharing and interoperability among different healthcare stakeholders are critical to realizing the full potential of digital health technologies. Interoperable systems, data standards, and standardized protocols are essential for accessible and comprehensive patient records. All facilitate coordinated care and support decision-making based on all available patient data, not just a portion of the data. An ecosystem that provides access to a patient's records no matter where the patient may go for service improves the quality of care and enhances patient safety, reducing the risk of medical errors and eliminating duplicative tests.

As with anything done in healthcare, there are ethical considerations with the adaptation of digital health technologies. There is the need to address data privacy, security, and the responsible use of AI including algorithmic bias. Ensuring that digital health technologies are accessible to all, regardless of income level, geographic region, or other social determinants of health, is crucial to achieving global health equity. Digital health solutions must prioritize the protection of patients' rights and foster fairness.

Collaboration should include all entities in the healthcare ecosystem. This includes healthcare providers, technology companies, policymakers, payers, pharmacy/life science companies, caregivers and others. Working together, these stakeholders have the ability to share knowledge, foster innovation, and develop solutions that address the difficult challenges in healthcare ecosystem. Novel initiatives from this inclusive band of stakeholders can lead to broad adoption of digital health technologies which can result in positive impacts on the quality and efficiency of healthcare delivery.

Collaborative efforts can facilitate sharing of best practices and lessons learned, leading to continuous learning environments that deliver the best possible outcomes for patients, empower providers, and enhance the overall efficiency and effectiveness of healthcare delivery. Digital healthcare transformation is powered by digital technologies that are interconnected, data-driven, and patient-centered. Global collaboration and knowledge sharing are key features allowing the advancement of digital health transformation and the realization of its full potential.

Digital health transformation provides us with an opportunity to make a fundamental shift in how we approach healthcare. The innovations discussed in this book are paving the way for a more connected, efficient, and patient-centered healthcare system. By embracing these advancements, we can look forward to a future where health outcomes are improved, disparities are reduced, and every person has the opportunity to lead a healthier life. We hope this book inspires you to be a part of this exciting journey and to contribute to the ongoing transformation of healthcare through digital technology.

Jay Spitulnik
Director, MS in Health Informatics Program,
Northeastern University, USA

Marie Maloney
Associate Director, MS in Health Informatics Program,
Northeastern University, USA

About the Editor

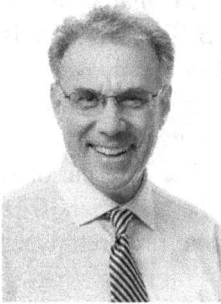

Dr. Jay Liebowitz served as the Professor of Business Innovation and Industry Transformation and Director of the AI-EDGE Center in the Crummer Graduate School of Business at Rollins College, as of August 2024. He now advises Thomas Jefferson University in their new programs in analytics and AI. He has recently served as the inaugural Executive-in-Residence for Public Service at Columbia University's Data Science Institute. He was previously a Visiting Professor at the Stillman School of Business and the MS-Business Analytics Capstone and Co-Program Director (External Relations) at Seton Hall University. He previously served as the Distinguished Chair of Applied Business and Finance at Harrisburg University of Science and Technology. Before HU, he was the Orkand Endowed Chair of Management and Technology in the Graduate School at the University of Maryland University College (UMUC). He served as a Full Professor in the Carey Business School at Johns Hopkins University. He was ranked one of the top 10 knowledge management researchers/practitioners out of 11,000 worldwide and was ranked #2 in KM Strategy worldwide according to the January 2010 *Journal of Knowledge Management*. At Johns Hopkins University, he was the founding Program Director for the Graduate Certificate in Competitive Intelligence and the Capstone Director of the MS-Information and Telecommunications Systems for Business Program, where he engaged over 30 organizations in industry, government, and not-for-profits in capstone projects.

Prior to joining Hopkins, Liebowitz was the first Knowledge Management Officer at NASA Goddard Space Flight Center. Before NASA, Liebowitz was the Robert W. Deutsch Distinguished Professor of Information Systems at the University of Maryland-Baltimore County, Professor of Management Science at George Washington University, and Chair of Artificial Intelligence at the U.S. Army War College.

Liebowitz is the Founding Editor-in-Chief of *Expert Systems With Applications: An International Journal* (published by Elsevier; ranked as a top-tier journal; Thomson Impact Factor from June 2021 is 8.665). He is a Fulbright Scholar, IEEE-USA Federal Communications Commission Executive Fellow, and Computer Educator of the Year (International Association for Computer Information Systems). He has published over 45 books and a myriad of journal articles on knowledge management, analytics, financial literacy, intelligent systems, and IT management. Liebowitz served as the Editor-in-Chief of *Procedia-CS* (Elsevier). He is also the Series Book Editor of the *Data Analytics Applications* book series (Taylor & Francis), as well as the Series Book Editor of the *Digital Transformation: Accelerating Organizational Intelligence* book series (World Scientific Publishing). In October 2011, the International Association for Computer Information Systems named the "Jay Liebowitz Outstanding Student Research Award" for the best student research paper at the IACIS Annual Conference. Liebowitz was the Fulbright Visiting Research Chair in Business at Queen's University for the Summer 2017 and a Fulbright Specialist at Dalarna University in Sweden in May 2019. He is in the top 2% of the top scientists in the world, according to a 2019 Stanford Study. As of 2021, he is the Visiting Distinguished Professor at the International School for Social and Business Studies in Slovenia. His recent books are as follows: *Data Analytics and AI* (Taylor & Francis, 2021), *The Business of Pandemics: The COVID-19 Story* (Taylor & Francis, 2021), *A Research Agenda for Knowledge Management and Analytics* (Elgar Publishers, 2021), *Online Learning Analytics* (Taylor & Francis, 2022), *Digital Transformation for the University of the Future* (World Scientific, 2022), *Cryptocurrency Concepts, Technology, and Applications* (Taylor & Francis, April 2023), *Pivoting Government Through Digital Transformation* (Taylor & Francis, 2024), and *Developing the Intuitive Executive: Using Analytics and Intuition for Success* (Taylor & Francis, 2024). His newest book, *Regulating Hate Speech Created by Generative AI*, was published by Taylor and Francis in August 2024. He has lectured and consulted worldwide.

List of Contributors

Richard James Boyd
CEO, UltiSim, USA

Leonardo Caporarello
Associate Dean for Online Learning, SDA Bocconi School of Management; Bocconi University, Italy

Alexeis Garcia Perez
Professor of Digital Business and Society, Aston Business School, Aston University, Birmingham, UK

Frank L. Gardner
Associate Dean for Academic Affairs, School of Health Sciences, Touro University, USA

McKenzie Gelvin
Touro University, USA

Sydney Harfenist
Touro University, USA

David M. Liebovitz, MD
Co-Director, Institute for Augmented Intelligence in Medicine – Center for Medical Education in Data Science and Digital Health; Associate Vice Chair for Clinical Informatics, Department of Medicine; Northwestern University Feinberg School of Medicine, USA

Steven Lorenzet
Dean, School of Health Sciences, Touro University, USA

Zella E. Moore
Professor of Psychology, Touro University, USA

Francesco Santarsiero
Professor, Università degli Studi della Basilicata, Italy

Paul Schmitter
Lecturer and Researcher, ZHAW School of Life Sciences and Facility Management, Switzerland

Iuliia Trabskaia
Academic Fellow, Bocconi University, Italy

Ingrid Vasiliu-Feltes, MD
Professor of Healthcare Informatics, Harrisburg University of Science and Technology, Harrisburg, PA, USA

Anne Wagner
Associate Professor, University of Lille, France

Contents

Chapter 1

Advancing Healthcare Transformation through Deep Tech: An Examination of Latest Trends, Challenges, and Opportunities

Ingrid Vasiliu-Feltes

Harrisburg University of Science and Technology,
Harrisburg, PA, USA

1. Introduction

The healthcare sector is undergoing a profound transformation, enabled by the confluence of advanced digital technologies and evolving scientific methodologies. This digital transformation is characterized by the systematic integration of cutting-edge technologies aimed at enhancing the quality, efficiency, and accessibility of healthcare services, fundamentally reshaping traditional paradigms of care delivery, administration, and patient interaction. At the core of this transformation lies a concerted effort to address entrenched challenges such as escalating operational costs, the demand for precision medicine, compliance with complex regulatory frameworks, and the imperative for seamless interoperability across diverse healthcare systems. Nevertheless, the accelerated pace of innovation introduces multidimensional complexities, requiring healthcare stakeholders – including providers, payers, regulatory bodies, and patients – to navigate an intricate landscape of legal, ethical, and operational imperatives.

Emerging technologies such as artificial intelligence (AI), blockchain, digital twin systems, multicloud computing, and anticipated 6G networks signify a radical shift in the healthcare sector. AI's capacity for processing and analyzing extensive datasets in real time facilitates advancements in predictive diagnostics, personalized therapeutic interventions, and large-scale epidemiological studies. Blockchain technology, with its decentralized and immutable architecture, ensures data integrity and security, thus fostering confidence in digital health infrastructures. Digital twins, or virtualized simulations of physical systems, support real-time decision-making processes, enhancing clinical training and patient-specific modeling, while multicloud and edge computing enable unprecedented levels of data accessibility and interoperability across complex healthcare ecosystems. Wearable devices, sensors, and bioimplant technologies offer the potential for continuous, real-time health monitoring, generating actionable data that can inform individualized care strategies. Complementary advances such as federated learning – enabling secure cross-institutional collaboration without compromising privacy – and data mesh and data fabric architectures enhance the resilience, scalability, and governance of healthcare data ecosystems.

This transformation, however, is not without challenges. Cybersecurity vulnerabilities and data privacy concerns remain persistent, while ethical considerations surrounding digital health solutions necessitate frameworks that safeguard patient autonomy and data integrity. Furthermore, the integration of complex, interdependent technologies – often referred to as deep tech orchestration – presents significant operational challenges. Nevertheless, digital transformation in healthcare presents substantial opportunities to advance diversity, equity, and inclusion (DEI) and environmental, social, and governance (ESG) goals. Aligning these transformative initiatives with DEI and ESG principles can foster inclusive, resilient, and sustainable healthcare models, benefiting diverse populations and contributing to global health equity.

This chapter provides a comprehensive analysis of the digital transformation landscape in healthcare, examining legal and regulatory frameworks, investment trajectories, and technological advancements. Additionally, it addresses the operational and ethical challenges that accompany digital health integration while highlighting opportunities to align healthcare transformations with DEI and ESG imperatives.

Ultimately, digital transformation holds the promise of creating a healthcare ecosystem that is more efficient, patient-centered, and resilient.

2. Global Landscape

2.1. *Legal and regulatory frameworks trends*

With the growing adoption of digital technologies in healthcare, legal and regulatory frameworks are evolving to address the complexities associated with data privacy, patient security, and operational transparency. Globally, governments and regulatory bodies are instituting laws and guidelines to manage healthcare data, including the Health Insurance Portability and Accountability Act (HIPAA) in the United States, the General Data Protection Regulation (GDPR) in the European Union, and other jurisdiction-specific regulations that impact digital health innovation. Legal frameworks surrounding telemedicine, wearable health devices, and data-sharing agreements are likewise advancing. Key trends in regulatory frameworks focus on standardizing interoperability, managing data exchange protocols, and strengthening consent mechanisms to ensure ethical and equitable utilization of digital health tools.

2.2. *Investment trends*

Investment in digital healthcare transformation has surged, driven by both public and private sectors recognizing its potential to optimize patient outcomes and operational efficiencies. Health technology startups attract substantial venture capital investment, while government grants support research in telemedicine and AI-driven diagnostics. Healthcare institutions are increasingly prioritizing investments in infrastructure, cybersecurity, and data governance to ensure compliance with evolving regulations and enhance data resilience. Investment patterns reflect a clear preference for cloud-native, scalable solutions that provide flexibility and facilitate adaptation to shifting market demands.

2.3. *Technology trends*

AI: The adoption of AI within healthcare is transformative, with machine learning algorithms enhancing diagnostic accuracy and enabling personalized therapeutics. Advanced algorithms, including convolutional

neural networks and generative adversarial networks, facilitate sophisticated analyses of multimodal datasets, supporting real-time decision-
making and predictive modeling.

Blockchain technology: Blockchain's decentralized architecture underpins
secure and immutable record-keeping. In healthcare, this facilitates
tamper-resistant patient records, traceability in pharmaceutical supply
chains, and secure data transactions, all crucial for maintaining trust in
digital health ecosystems.

Digital twins: Digital twin technology, which involves the creation of
virtualized replicas of physical systems, allows for dynamic simulations
of patient conditions. This technology facilitates precision medicine by
enabling clinicians to model treatment outcomes based on individual
patient characteristics, thus optimizing therapeutic strategies.

Multicloud computing: Multicloud architectures provide a robust infrastructure for healthcare data management, supporting scalability and fault
tolerance. By distributing data processing and storage across multiple
cloud providers, multicloud solutions enhance resilience against service
disruptions and data latency issues.

Edge computing: Edge computing enables localized data processing,
which is critical for latency-sensitive applications such as intensive
care monitoring and remote diagnostics. By positioning computational
resources near the data source, edge computing facilitates real-time analytics and responsive decision-making in clinical environments.

Federated learning: Federated learning enables decentralized machine
learning, allowing healthcare institutions to derive insights from aggregated
datasets while preserving patient privacy. This approach is particularly
advantageous in collaborative research settings, where sensitive data must
be securely shared across institutions.

Data mesh and data fabric architectures: Data mesh and data fabric
frameworks facilitate decentralized data management, supporting scalability, resilience, and data democratization within healthcare systems.
These architectures allow healthcare organizations to integrate, manage,

and utilize disparate datasets effectively, enabling a more agile response to healthcare demands.

Wearable devices and sensors: Wearable health technology empowers continuous monitoring of vital health metrics, generating longitudinal data that supports preventative care and early intervention. These devices, often equipped with advanced sensors, transmit real-time data to clinicians, enabling proactive healthcare management.

Bioimplants: Bioimplants, comprising sensors and actuators, provide a direct interface between physiological systems and digital health platforms. These devices enable real-time monitoring of critical health metrics and can facilitate targeted therapeutic delivery, exemplifying a transformative approach to patient care.

Satellite internet and 6G connectivity: Advanced connectivity solutions such as satellite internet and anticipated 6G networks are poised to address healthcare access disparities in underserved areas, enabling seamless, high-speed data exchange across remote healthcare facilities.

3. Challenges

3.1. *Cybersecurity*

The digital transformation of healthcare inherently increases exposure to cyber threats, necessitating robust and adaptive cybersecurity measures. Protecting patient data from malicious attacks such as ransomware and unauthorized access requires a comprehensive approach that encompasses encryption, anomaly detection, and intrusion prevention systems.

3.2. *Digital ethics*

Ethical considerations surrounding digital health focus on maintaining patient privacy, autonomy, and data integrity. Digital ethics frameworks are essential to guide healthcare organizations in the responsible deployment of digital technologies, ensuring transparency and accountability in data utilization.

3.3. *Deep tech orchestration*

The orchestration of complex technological systems within healthcare presents significant challenges, often involving the integration of heterogeneous data sources, applications, and platforms. Deep tech orchestration requires sophisticated governance structures to ensure interoperability, standardization, and operational coherence across advanced healthcare solutions.

4. Opportunities

4.1. *Alignment with DEI*

Digital transformation provides an avenue to promote DEI within healthcare by increasing accessibility to underserved populations and addressing systemic health disparities. Technologies that support telemedicine and mobile health initiatives enable healthcare providers to reach a broader demographic, contributing to equitable health outcomes.

4.2. *ESG*

The integration of digital technologies presents opportunities to advance ESG goals within healthcare, enhancing transparency in resource allocation, minimizing environmental impact, and fostering sustainable healthcare practices. Blockchain and AI-driven analytics can provide insights into supply chain efficiency, contributing to environmentally responsible healthcare operations.

5. Future Directions for Research and Development

The future of healthcare is set to be transformed by technologies, such as Web 3.0, the healthcare metaverse, and an industrial healthcare omniverse. Together, these advancements hold the potential to reshape patient care, medical research, and the way healthcare providers collaborate globally, moving us toward a more integrated, secure, and efficient system.

5.1. *Web 3.0 in healthcare*

Web 3.0, or the "semantic web," introduces a new level of connectivity and data ownership that holds immense promise for healthcare. With blockchain technology at its core, Web 3.0 enables decentralized data storage, allowing patients and healthcare providers to manage and share data more securely and transparently. Instead of centralized databases, patient data could be stored on decentralized networks, giving patients more control over who accesses their health information. This could mitigate privacy concerns while enabling seamless data sharing across providers, improving continuity of care, especially for patients with chronic conditions or those who frequently relocate.

Furthermore, Web 3.0's blockchain technology can enable "smart contracts" within healthcare settings. These contracts could automatically enforce certain terms and conditions, such as verifying insurance coverage or facilitating automated payments once services are rendered, reducing administrative overhead and increasing the speed and efficiency of trans- actions. As a result, the patient experience can be streamlined, and provid- ers can focus more on delivering care than managing paperwork. In addition, Web 3.0 could open the door to decentralized autonomous organizations (DAOs) in healthcare, where stakeholders collaboratively manage healthcare funds, research grants, or community health initiatives in a transparent and community-driven way.

5.2. *The healthcare metaverse*

The concept of a healthcare metaverse brings with it a digital environment where patients, doctors, and researchers can interact in immersive ways. In the healthcare metaverse, virtual spaces will allow for remote consulta- tions, therapy sessions, and even surgical simulations. Patients could have consultations with specialists from around the world without leaving their homes, a boon for those in remote or underserved areas. With advanced VR (Virtual Reality) and AR (Augmented Reality) tools, doctors can vir- tually examine patients, visualize complex surgical procedures in 3D, or use simulations for training purposes.

For mental health, the healthcare metaverse offers particularly excit- ing applications. Therapeutic environments can be crafted in virtual spaces to help patients confront fears or process trauma in controlled, immersive ways. Group therapy sessions or support groups could also be conducted virtually, offering social support without geographic limitations.

Additionally, the metaverse can serve as a platform for healthcare education and training. Medical students and professionals can practice procedures in a safe, simulated environment, enhancing their skills and reducing the risk of errors in real-life scenarios. Through these immersive, interactive experiences, the metaverse can contribute to a higher standard of care.

5.3. *The industrial healthcare omniverse*

Beyond individual patient care, the industrial healthcare omniverse represents a broader digital ecosystem where healthcare providers, manufacturers, and suppliers interact in a highly connected way. In this omniverse, medical supply chains, manufacturing, research labs, and healthcare institutions can coordinate in real time, facilitating a rapid response to demand fluctuations, disease outbreaks, or supply shortages. The industrial healthcare omniverse could integrate digital twins – digital replicas of physical assets, processes, or systems – of everything from hospital equipment to entire medical facilities, allowing for predictive maintenance and optimized resource allocation. Imagine a scenario where a hospital needs additional ventilators during a health crisis. With digital twins and connected systems, manufacturers could receive real-time data on the hospital's needs and adjust their production accordingly, significantly reducing lead times. This level of integration would also enable hospitals to conduct more accurate forecasting and planning, preparing for patient influxes or anticipating equipment needs based on data insights.

Through these interwoven platforms, the omniverse will enable more collaborative research and innovation. Pharmaceutical companies, research institutions, and clinicians can work together within shared virtual labs, running simulations and sharing findings instantaneously, accelerating the pace of medical discovery.

6. Conclusion

The digital transformation of healthcare is redefining the healthcare landscape, offering unprecedented capabilities to enhance diagnostic precision, treatment efficacy, and overall patient engagement. This transformation requires a comprehensive understanding of the legal and regulatory frameworks, investment trends, and emerging technologies shaping the industry. However, as healthcare organizations adopt these innovations, they must address inherent challenges, including cybersecurity risks, ethical dilemmas, and the complexity of deep tech orchestration. These challenges necessitate a proactive, interdisciplinary approach to balance the drive for technological innovation with the ethical imperative of patient safety and data security.

Notwithstanding these challenges, the digital transformation of healthcare presents significant opportunities to advance DEI and ESG principles, fostering a more inclusive and sustainable healthcare ecosystem. By aligning digital health initiatives with DEI and ESG objectives, healthcare organizations not only enhance operational efficiency but also generate societal value, advancing health equity and environmental stewardship.

As healthcare continues its trajectory toward digital transformation, a coordinated effort among stakeholders – including policymakers, healthcare providers, technology developers, and patients – will be essential to ensure a future where digital technology augments, rather than detracts from, the core values of human-centered healthcare. Guided by responsible innovation principles, digital transformation has the potential to create a more resilient, efficient, and patient-centric healthcare system, ultimately contributing to improved global health outcomes and equitable access to care.

References

Abi Saad, E., Tremblay, N., and Agogué, M. (2024). A multi-level perspective on innovation intermediaries: The case of the diffusion of digital technologies in healthcare. *Technovation, 129*, 102899.

Bevere, D. and Faccilongo, N. (2024). Shaping the future of healthcare: Integrating ecology and digital innovation. *Sustainability, 16*(9), 3835.

Darda, P. and Matta, N. (2024). The nexus of healthcare and technology: A thematic analysis of digital transformation through artificial intelligence. In *Transformative Approaches to Patient Literacy and Healthcare Innovation*, pp. 261–282. IGI Global.

Hulsen, T. (2024). Applications of the metaverse in medicine and healthcare. *Advances in Laboratory Medicine/Avances en Medicina de Laboratorio, 5*(2), 159–165.

Kumari, D., Sharma, S., Chawla, M., and Panda, S. (2024). A manifesto for healthcare based blockchain: Research directions for the future generation. *Journal of the Institution of Engineers (India): Series B*, 1–22.

Li, Y., Gunasekeran, D. V., RaviChandran, N., Tan, T. F., Ong, J. C. L., Thirunavukarasu, A. J., Polascik, B. W., Habash, R., Khaderi, K., and Ting, D. S. W. (2024). The next generation of healthcare ecosystem in the metaverse. *Biomedical Journal, 47*(3), 100679.

Martin, M. S. and Alarcón-Urbistondo, P. (2024). Digital transformation in healthcare and medical practices: Advancements, challenges, and future opportunities. In *Emerging Technologies for Health Literacy and Medical Practice*, pp. 176–197. IGI Global.

Shardeo, V., Sarkar, B. D., Mir, U. B., and Kaushik, P. (2024). Adoption of metaverse in healthcare sector: An empirical analysis of its enablers. *IEEE Transactions on Engineering Management*, 1–15.

Swan, E. L., Peltier, J. W., and Dahl, A. J. (2024). Artificial intelligence in healthcare: The value co-creation process and influence of other digital health transformations. *Journal of Research in Interactive Marketing*, *18*(1), 109–126.

Ullah, S., Li, J., Chen, J., ALI, I., Khan, S., Ahad, A., Ullah, F., and Leung, V. C. M. (2024). A survey on emerging trends and applications of 5G and 6G to healthcare environments. *ACM Computing Surveys, 57*(4), 3703154.

Wong, B. K. M., Vengusamy, S., and Bastrygina, T. (2024). Healthcare digital transformation through the adoption of artificial intelligence. In *Artificial Intelligence, Big Data, Blockchain and 5G for the Digital Transformation of the Healthcare Industry*, pp. 87–110. Academic Press.

Chapter 2

Overcoming Challenges in Healthcare Digital Transformation: The Innovation Lab Approach

Francesco Santarsiero

Università degli Studi della Basilicata, Italy

1. Introduction

Nowadays, the healthcare sector stands at a critical juncture, shaped by evolving demographic trends, escalating patient expectations, and an imperative to optimize public spending. The lessons of the COVID-19 pandemic have left a profound impact, accelerating the adoption of digital technologies while exposing deep-seated systemic weaknesses. As the focus shifts from crisis response to building resilient and sustainable healthcare systems, the role of digital transformation (DT) has become increasingly central (Dal Mas *et al.*, 2023). DT is not just a technological upgrade; it represents a comprehensive rethinking of how healthcare services are delivered, with an emphasis on efficiency, accessibility, and patient-centricity.

However, achieving effective DT in healthcare remains a formidable challenge (Dionisio *et al.*, 2022; Santarsiero *et al.*, 2023). High investment costs, lengthy development cycles, regulatory hurdles, and cultural resistance frequently hinder progress. Unlike other sectors, where lean methodologies and rapid prototyping enable quick iterations, healthcare often relies on prolonged research and development phases conducted in isolated environments. This disconnect between innovation processes and real-world applications can lead to solutions that fail to address the actual needs of patients and stakeholders. Moreover, the fragmentation of healthcare ecosystems exacerbates these challenges, creating silos that impede collaboration and knowledge sharing (Limna, 2023).

The transition to a digitally enabled healthcare system requires more than just new technologies. It demands a fundamental shift in mindset across organizations and stakeholders (Raimo *et al.*, 2022). Patients, healthcare providers, policymakers, and innovators must work collaboratively to design solutions that are not only technologically advanced but also practical, inclusive, and aligned with real-world demands. The principles of open innovation and co-creation offer a pathway to overcome these barriers by fostering ecosystems where diverse actors contribute to the innovation process and share its risks and rewards. These approaches ensure that innovation is not only driven by technology but also shaped by the lived experiences and insights of end users (Agarwal *et al.*, 2010).

In this context, Innovation Labs have emerged as a promising approach to addressing the complexities of healthcare DT (Santarsiero *et al.*, 2023). These labs serve as platforms for experimentation, bringing together multidisciplinary teams to ideate, prototype, and test solutions in controlled yet realistic settings. Whether physical, virtual, or hybrid, Innovation Labs create environments where collaboration, creativity, and user-centered design are prioritized. By acting as testbeds for emerging technologies and methodologies, they reduce the risks and costs traditionally associated with healthcare innovation while enhancing the relevance and scalability of new solutions.

Despite their significant potential, the adoption and implementation of Innovation Labs in healthcare remain limited. Key questions persist regarding their effectiveness in addressing sector-specific challenges, including stringent regulatory constraints, concerns over patient data privacy, and the complexities of integrating innovations into existing clinical workflows. Gaining a deeper understanding of how these labs can serve as catalysts for digital transformation is essential to unlocking their full potential and addressing the pressing and evolving needs of the healthcare sector.

This chapter adopts a mixed-method approach to bridge this gap. It combines a review of recent literature on healthcare DT with case examples of Innovation Labs, examining how these labs address contemporary challenges and align with emerging trends in innovation management. The primary objectives are to identify the barriers to successful DT, explore the role of Innovation Labs as platforms for innovation and experimentation, and provide actionable insights and strategies for their implementation and management.

The research questions guiding this analysis are as follows: (1) *What are the most pressing challenges in achieving successful digital transformation in healthcare, and how have they evolved in recent years?* (2) *How can Innovation Labs enable healthcare organizations to overcome these challenges and drive effective digital transformation?*

By answering these questions, this chapter aims to deepen theoretical and practical understanding of how Innovation Labs can catalyze healthcare DT. It provides insights into their structure, functioning, and management, highlighting best practices and tools for fostering innovation. The findings offer valuable guidance for healthcare organizations, policymakers, and innovators seeking to harness the transformative potential of Innovation Labs in shaping the future of healthcare.

2. Digital Transformation in Healthcare: Dimensions, Challenges, and Opportunities

2.1. *Dimensions of digital transformation in healthcare*

DT in healthcare is reshaping how medical services are designed, delivered, and experienced, heralding a new era of efficiency, accessibility, and patient-centered care. At its core, DT integrates advanced digital technologies – such as Artificial Intelligence (AI), Big Data analytics, Internet of Things (IoT), telemedicine platforms, and wearable devices – into healthcare workflows. These technologies collectively enable real-time clinical decision-making, predictive analytics, and improved patient outcomes, reflecting a broader societal trend toward personalization and digital empowerment (Al-haimi *et al.*, 2021; Schiuma *et al.*, 2021).

Central to DT in healthcare is the strategic implementation of digital tools that profoundly reshape organizational behaviors and knowledge dynamics. The integration of emerging technologies into routine healthcare operations not only enhances efficiency but also fosters dynamic knowledge creation and management processes (Limna, 2022). These advancements enable healthcare professionals to shift from repetitive, time-intensive tasks to high-value activities that directly influence patient outcomes. This transition is instrumental in driving business model innovation, equipping organizations with the flexibility and agility required to navigate the evolving demands and challenges of the healthcare sector (Schiuma *et al.*, 2021).

The COVID-19 pandemic served as a critical accelerant for DT in healthcare, underscoring the indispensable role of digital technologies in maintaining service continuity amidst unprecedented challenges (Peek *et al.*, 2023). During this period, tools such as telemedicine platforms and remote monitoring systems became vital, especially for populations in remote or underserved areas. These innovations facilitated virtual consultations, real-time patient monitoring, and efficient information sharing, thereby mitigating risks associated with in-person interactions and ensuring sustained access to essential medical services (Li *et al.*, 2016).

The pandemic also exposed systemic weaknesses, including fragmented information systems and poor interoperability, which impeded seamless data exchange and collaboration across healthcare networks. These vulnerabilities catalyzed targeted investments and reforms, aimed at building more robust and resilient healthcare infrastructures. The swift adoption of digital solutions during the crisis not only addressed immediate public health needs but also highlighted the strategic importance of integrating these technologies into standard practice (Dash, 2020). The continued reliance on telemedicine, remote monitoring, and other digital tools in the post-pandemic era reflects an industry-wide recognition of their potential to enhance adaptability, resilience, and efficiency in healthcare systems (Dal Mas *et al.*, 2023; Peek *et al.*, 2023).

DT has significantly advanced *operational efficiencies* in healthcare, elevating both the quality and accessibility of care. A key driver of this transformation is the automation of labor-intensive administrative processes, which optimizes resource allocation and streamlines workflows. Technologies such as AI and data analytics are central to this evolution, providing actionable insights from complex datasets to support clinical decision-making. For example, IoT-enabled devices facilitate seamless data exchange across care settings, improving treatment coordination while reducing redundancies (Gopal *et al.*, 2019; Schiuma *et al.*, 2021). Similarly, cloud-based platforms enable secure storage and analysis of large-scale datasets, which can be utilized to identify trends, predict disease outbreaks, and develop targeted interventions. These innovations not only save time but also enhance patient outcomes by fostering evidence-based practices and enabling a proactive approach to health management (Raimo *et al.*, 2022).

Moreover, the widespread adoption of electronic health records (EHRs) has facilitated seamless information exchange across healthcare networks, reducing inefficiencies and enabling better provider coordination (Dioniso *et al.*, 2022). Predictive analytics, underpinned by big data, further supports early disease detection and enhances diagnostic accuracy, laying a solid foundation for preventive care initiatives.

Operational processes within healthcare organizations have undergone profound transformation due to the adoption of digital tools (Gopal *et al.*, 2019). Telemedicine applications, for instance, have expanded clinical services to underserved and rural regions, effectively addressing disparities in healthcare access. These platforms enable remote diagnostics and consultation, ensuring that patients in isolated areas receive timely and effective care. By bridging gaps in infrastructure and resources, these advancements also help mitigate social inequities by lowering the financial barriers typically associated with traditional healthcare delivery (Agarwal *et al.*, 2010; Hermann *et al.*, 2017; Khodadad-Saryazdi, 2021).

Beyond patient-facing services, DT has significantly impacted the healthcare *workforce*. Automation of routine operations enables healthcare professionals to dedicate more time to value-added activities, such as patient engagement and care planning. Collaboration tools, such as video conferencing and shared digital workspaces, enhance productivity by promoting knowledge sharing and fostering team-based approaches to care delivery. Additionally, the integration of data into decision-making systems empowers organizations to adopt data-driven management strategies, improving both clinical outcomes and operational efficiency (Sousa *et al.*, 2019).

The convergence of these technological advancements underscores DT's broader value proposition in healthcare: the ability to deliver high-quality, patient-centered care while optimizing resource utilization and addressing systemic inefficiencies. As digital innovations continue to evolve, they illuminate the critical need for building digital infrastructures that are both effective and equitable. Ensuring universal accessibility to these benefits is paramount for addressing persistent healthcare disparities and fostering an inclusive, innovation-driven ecosystem.

DT is also redefining the *patient experience* by fostering interactive, personalized, and empowering care journeys. Patients are now active participants in their healthcare, supported by wearable technologies, mobile health applications, and telehealth platforms that provide real-time insights into their health conditions. This patient-centric model enables informed decision-making, preventive care, and effective chronic disease management (Kraus *et al.*, 2021; Laurenza *et al.*, 2018).

Data analytics plays a pivotal role in understanding patient behaviors, preferences, and needs, allowing for highly personalized care delivery. Digital platforms enhance communication between patients and healthcare providers, fostering a collaborative relationship that improves adherence to treatment plans and strengthens trust. For instance, AI-driven diagnostics integrated with patient health histories enable the customization of treatment plans, demonstrating how DT merges technological advancements with human-centered care (Dash, 2020).

Furthermore, the integration of digital technologies has also revolutionized healthcare *business models*, creating new pathways for value creation and service delivery. Subscription-based telehealth services, virtual pharmacies, and AI-driven diagnostic tools enable healthcare providers to diversify their offerings while aligning financial sustainability with improved patient outcomes (Kraus *et al.*, 2021; Nambisan, 2017). Blockchain technology enhances trust and transparency by securing sensitive patient records and ensuring compliant data sharing among stakeholders (Santarsiero *et al.*, 2023).

Emerging business models also reflect the dynamic potential of DT. Organizations leverage digital globalization to optimize services and reach underserved populations while maintaining high standards of care. These innovations highlight how technological integration reshapes value creation, capturing economic and societal benefits alike (Nambisan, 2017).

2.2. *Challenges and opportunities in healthcare digital transformation*

Despite its transformative potential, DT in healthcare faces several barriers that hinder its scalability and impact. Fragmented information systems and the lack of interoperability across platforms obstruct seamless data exchange, while regulatory constraints often slow down the adoption of innovative technologies. Resistance to change among healthcare professionals – driven by insufficient training, limited digital literacy, and fear of increased workload – further exacerbates these challenges. Addressing these issues requires targeted workforce development programs, structured training initiatives, and clear demonstrations of the tangible benefits of digital tools (Agarwal *et al.*, 2010; Hermes *et al.*, 2020; Kakale, 2024).

Data privacy, cybersecurity, and regulatory concerns are particularly pronounced, as the widespread digitization of sensitive patient records increases exposure to breaches and unauthorized access (Kraus *et al.*, 2021). Robust security protocols, such as encryption, multifactor authentication, and transparent governance frameworks, are essential to building trust and ensuring compliance (Kakale, 2024). Economic disparities further complicate DT adoption, with low-income and underserved regions often lacking the necessary infrastructure, funding, and expertise. Bridging this digital divide requires government subsidies, innovative service delivery models, and targeted investments in infrastructure (Khodadad-Saryazdi, 2021).

The high costs associated with DT also deter its widespread adoption. Many healthcare organizations perceive DT initiatives as prohibitively expensive, especially when the return on investment is not immediately apparent. Smaller institutions and those operating in resource-constrained environments are particularly affected by this perception. Demonstrating the long-term benefits of DT, including cost savings from reduced hospital stays and improved operational efficiency, is critical to securing investment and fostering adoption (Agarwal *et al.*, 2010; Hermes *et al.*, 2020).

Insufficient digital skills among healthcare professionals present another challenge. The successful implementation of DT relies on a workforce capable of leveraging advanced technologies, such as artificial intelligence, data analytics, and cybersecurity systems. Workforce development programs, partnerships with academic institutions, and continuing education initiatives are critical to addressing this gap. Without adequately trained personnel, the adoption of digital technologies risks being suboptimal, undermining their potential impact (Sousa *et al.*, 2019).

Organizational silos and entrenched operational barriers further hinder the integration of DT in healthcare. Many organizations operate with fragmented communication and limited collaboration between departments and stakeholders. This lack of cohesion undermines the effectiveness of DT initiatives, as it prevents the holistic implementation of digital tools. Creating cross-functional teams, fostering a collaborative culture, and utilizing innovation labs to break down silos can significantly enhance integration efforts and maximize the value of DT (Kane *et al.*, 2021).

Ensuring accessibility and equity in digital healthcare solutions is another pressing challenge. Digital tools must be inclusive, addressing the needs of populations in remote areas or with limited digital literacy. Designing user-friendly platforms, simplifying interfaces, and providing training programs for patients and healthcare providers can help address these disparities. Equity-focused approaches are crucial to ensuring that DT serves as a bridge rather than a barrier, helping to close gaps in healthcare delivery rather than exacerbating them (Shaw *et al.*, 2024).

Despite these barriers, the opportunities presented by DT in healthcare are substantial. Interoperable platforms and standardized data-sharing protocols offer a pathway to streamlined care delivery and improved collaboration among providers. Open innovation frameworks, which engage diverse stakeholders – including startups, clinicians, patients, and policymakers – can foster co-designed solutions tailored to the specific needs of healthcare ecosystems. Moreover, investments in digital skills development and workforce training can empower healthcare professionals to effectively utilize advanced technologies, ensuring their optimal impact.

As the following section on Innovation Labs demonstrates, these labs provide a robust framework for addressing many of these challenges. By acting as platforms for co-creation, experimentation, and stakeholder engagement, innovation labs can bridge gaps in digital adoption and drive sustainable transformation. The challenges identified here – ranging from interoperability and regulatory constraints to workforce skill gaps and organizational silos – can be systematically tackled through the structured approaches facilitated by innovation labs. Through case examples and evidence-based practices, the role of innovation labs as catalysts for overcoming barriers in healthcare DT will be explored, providing actionable insights into their transformative potential.

3. The Innovation Lab Approach

Innovation Labs have emerged as pivotal instruments for supporting organizations in their DT initiatives. These labs serve as dynamic environments that facilitate critical and creative thinking, providing organizations with the necessary resources, methodologies, and frameworks to foster a digital culture, implement technology-driven solutions, digitize operational processes, and cultivate sustainable pathways for innovation

(Santarsiero *et al.*, 2024). Their role in advancing DT has garnered increasing attention from both academia and industry practitioners, with a growing body of literature highlighting their potential to drive business model innovation across a variety of sectors (Fecher *et al.*, 2018; Trucker, 2017).

Innovation Labs are celebrated for their ability to catalyze innovation by creating environments conducive to experimentation, ideation, and the development of impactful solutions. They provide structured spaces where organizations can test novel ideas, address complex challenges, and prototype solutions before scaling them to broader applications. This capacity to serve as a testbed for innovation has solidified their reputation as transformative tools in contemporary management practices (Memon *et al.*, 2018; Schmidt *et al.*, 2015). The concept of the Innovation Lab was formally introduced in management studies to denote designated spaces aimed at enhancing an organization's ability to innovate by offering both physical and conceptual support for creative and strategic endeavors. Innovation Labs are purpose-built environments designed to foster ideation, experimentation, and the development of innovative solutions. Lewis and Moultrie (2005) characterize these labs as dedicated facilities aimed at encouraging creative behaviors and supporting innovative initiatives through the provision of essential tools and resources. Magadley and Birdy (2009) extend this perspective by emphasizing the role of creative environments in facilitating collaboration, allowing individuals to push beyond traditional constraints and explore novel approaches. These labs are often considered a defining feature of contemporary innovation practices, as they enable employees and stakeholders to collaboratively engage in the exploration of new ideas and solutions (Bloom and Faulkner, 2016; D'Auria *et al.*, 2017; Schmidt and Brinks, 2017).

The intrinsic connection between creative environments, organizational innovation, and performance has been further substantiated by Magadley and Birdi (2009), who position Innovation Labs as critical hubs for challenging conventional boundaries and driving impactful change. A distinguishing attribute of these labs is their ability to support open innovation, user-driven innovation, and collaborative innovation. They establish settings where hierarchical barriers are minimized, empowering diverse stakeholders – including employees, users, and external collaborators – to co-create solutions that address real-world challenges and align with stakeholder needs (Lewis and Moultrie, 2005; Memon *et al.*, 2018; Osorio *et al.*, 2019; Schmidt *et al.*, 2014).

Despite the emphasis on their physical and collaborative nature, scholars caution against reducing Innovation Labs to mere "innovation theatres," where activities are symbolic rather than substantive. To avoid such pitfalls, these labs must act as "innovation engines," aligning their initiatives with organizational strategies and employing robust methodologies to engage stakeholders meaningfully. This approach ensures that Innovation Labs contribute tangible value, driving satisfaction and organizational performance while maintaining their central role as catalysts for sustainable innovation (Bogers, 2018; De Silva *et al.*, 2019; Fecher *et al.*, 2018).

The emphasis on the physical structural component of Innovation Labs has diminished over time, primarily due to advancements in technology and shifts in competitive environments (Santarsiero *et al.*, 2024). Hybrid configurations of Innovation Labs, which combine physical and virtual elements, are gaining prominence by enabling remote services and fostering global collaboration. These configurations make it easier to engage with partners, experts, and stakeholders from diverse locations, thereby broadening the reach and scalability of activities such as training and ideation. Participants can now engage remotely, allowing Innovation Labs to transcend geographical boundaries and extend their influence to a wider audience.

Historically, the physical spaces of Innovation Labs were often perceived as showcase venues rather than functional innovation hubs. Managers frequently viewed these labs as isolated units where cutting-edge technologies were displayed, and innovation was confined to a select group of experts. This disconnection from the broader organization often resulted in innovations that were misunderstood or poorly integrated, leading to low adoption rates and increased risks of failure. Moreover, a closed approach to external collaboration sometimes produced solutions that did not align with market demands, further jeopardizing their success.

To address these limitations, the concept of Innovation Labs has evolved into a more relational and dynamic framework. Modern Innovation Labs are increasingly conceived as platforms that facilitate connections within their ecosystems, fostering open innovation and iterative learning with consumers and stakeholders. These labs are no longer limited to physical spaces but are instead viewed as hybrid environments – physical, virtual, and relational – designed to nurture an innovative organizational climate.

This reimagined approach positions Innovation Labs as strategic management initiatives that support creativity and innovation through user-driven and open innovation practices. They serve as hubs for engaging diverse stakeholders in collaborative innovation processes, gaining deeper insights into user needs, driving technological transformation, and identifying opportunities for value creation. By emphasizing flexibility and inclusivity, Innovation Labs now focus on delivering tangible business solutions that capture and deliver value while ensuring alignment with organizational goals and market demands.

Innovation Labs can be effectively conceptualized as comprehensive models of innovation management, characterized by three core dimensions. The first dimension, "atmosphere for innovation," involves creating an environment – whether physical, virtual, or hybrid – that is intentionally designed to foster interaction, creativity, and collaboration. This space serves as a catalyst for innovation by encouraging open communication, reducing hierarchical barriers, and enabling dynamic exchanges among participants.

The second dimension, "time for exploration," emphasizes the strategic allocation of time dedicated to activities, such as brainstorming, critical thinking, and creatively addressing complex challenges. This temporal flexibility allows individuals and teams to diverge from routine tasks and focus on generating and refining innovative ideas without the constraints of immediate deliverables or rigid deadlines.

The third dimension, "platform to experiment," encompasses the provision of tools, resources, and infrastructure necessary for prototyping and testing new ideas. This includes access to advanced technologies, expert facilitation, and feedback mechanisms that enable iterative development and risk mitigation. By offering a structured yet flexible platform for experimentation, Innovation Labs help bridge the gap between ideation and implementation.

Together, these dimensions create an integrated framework that allows organizations to embed innovation into their culture and processes seamlessly. By aligning creative efforts with strategic objectives, Innovation Labs enable the generation of innovative solutions that are not only feasible and scalable but also aligned with organizational and market needs (Santarsiero *et al.*, 2019; 2020; Lewis and Moultrie, 2005; Memon *et al.*, 2018; Osorio *et al.*, 2019). The operation of Innovation Labs is grounded in the principles of open innovation and continuous engagement. These labs promote user-driven approaches, facilitate stakeholder participation, and identify opportunities to address complex challenges. Acting as platforms for testing and experimentation, they provide structured environments where new ideas can be prototyped, refined through iterative feedback, and validated for broader implementation (Schiuma and Santarsiero, 2023). This structured methodology ensures that innovative initiatives are practical, resource-efficient, and aligned with real-world applications.

This evolved configuration of Innovation Labs makes them particularly advantageous for healthcare organizations, a sector defined by complex regulatory environments, diverse stakeholder needs, and the rapid evolution of medical technologies. Innovation Labs provide healthcare organizations with the structured environments needed to navigate these challenges, enabling the integration of emerging technologies with patient-centered care models. By fostering collaboration among patients, clinicians, policymakers, and technology developers, Innovation Labs create ecosystems where innovative ideas can be co-created, prototyped, and rigorously tested. This minimizes the risks associated with large-scale implementation and ensures that solutions are both technologically robust and responsive to patient needs.

The role of Innovation Labs as hubs for open innovation also aligns with the healthcare sector's need for continuous learning and adaptation. These labs support iterative learning processes, stakeholder engagement, and the integration of cutting-edge technologies to address critical challenges, such as interoperability, digital literacy, and equitable care delivery. By doing so, Innovation Labs act as essential enablers of DT in healthcare, advancing operational efficiency, enhancing patient outcomes, and fostering system-wide resilience.

Building on this understanding, the following section delves into the specific applications of Innovation Labs in healthcare, exploring case examples that illustrate their potential to address sector-specific challenges and catalyze transformative change.

4. Innovation Labs in Healthcare

Innovation Labs in healthcare represent transformative platforms designed to drive DT and foster innovation within a rapidly evolving sector (Molloy, 2018; Tasca *et al.*, 2019). By serving as collaborative spaces, these Labs bring together clinicians, researchers, patients, startups, and other stakeholders, creating an interdisciplinary ecosystem to address the unique challenges of healthcare. Anchored in principles of open innovation and co-creation, these Labs leverage cutting-edge digital technologies to generate solutions that not only respond to pressing healthcare needs but also reimagine how care is delivered and experienced (Torvinen and Jansson, 2023).

Structured often as public–private partnerships, Healthcare Innovation Labs pool resources and expertise from diverse sectors to enhance their operational and innovation capacities (Santarsiero *et al.*, 2023). Examples such as HealthHUB Finland and the D-HEALTH at the University of Southern California demonstrate the potential of these collaborations to secure funding from regional, national, and international sources (Tolomiczenko and Sanger, 2015). These funds support the development of advanced infrastructures that include open workspaces, state-of-the-art teamwork technologies, virtual and remote collaboration tools, and rapid prototyping equipment. Moreover, a strategic emphasis on inclusivity ensures that these Labs remain dynamic spaces where diverse perspectives converge to fuel creative and innovative processes.

Central to their mission is a user-driven approach that prioritizes the real-world needs of the communities they serve. For instance, the Healthcare Living Lab Catalonia (HCLLC) in Spain unites healthcare centers, technology hubs, and living labs to expedite the prototyping, testing, and validation of innovative solutions in real-world settings (Healthcare Living Lab Catalonia, 2024). Similarly, BETiC in India focuses on developing affordable medical devices tailored to local healthcare challenges (Ravi, 2020). These Labs begin their processes by identifying critical issues, forming interdisciplinary teams, and facilitating ideation, prototyping, and validation phases. Acting as incubators and accelerators, they support the creation of new healthcare products, services, and business models, fostering a culture of collaboration and innovation that extends beyond the Lab itself.

The physical and virtual infrastructures of these labs are meticulously designed to inspire creativity and flexibility. For example, the Hephaïstos FabLab at Bicêtre Hospital in France provides a space equipped with advanced fabrication tools, enabling healthcare professionals to prototype and test new medical devices (Scarmoncin *et al.*, 2022).

Functionally, Healthcare Innovation Labs offer a suite of services tailored to the specific challenges of digital healthcare transformation. The Digital Health Living Lab in the UK exemplifies this by co-creating digital health solutions through collaboration among academia, industry, and end-users, thereby accelerating the adoption of person-centered technologies (Fotis *et al.*, 2023). Additionally, the Innovations in International

Health initiative at MIT facilitated multidisciplinary research to develop medical technologies suitable for developing countries, emphasizing the importance of context-specific solutions (International Health Initiative, 2024).

These Labs also act as networking hubs, fostering knowledge exchange and collaboration. Networking and dissemination activities are integral to these labs, aiming to strengthen their ecosystems and attract new partnerships. BETiC, for example, organizes events such as the Medical Device Hackathon (MEDHA) and the Medical Device Innovation Camp (MEDIC) to bring together diverse participants, fostering collaboration and accelerating medical device innovation (Ravi, 2020). Similarly, the Healthcare Living Lab Catalonia connects SMEs and startups with healthcare providers to facilitate the rapid development and implementation of innovative solutions.

Management practices within these labs are aligned with the principles of open innovation and continuous learning. The Hephaïstos FabLab, for instance, operates within a hospital ecosystem, fostering innovation by providing services that support the development and implementation of new medical devices (Scarmoncin *et al.*, 2022).

Innovation Labs also tackle critical challenges in healthcare DT, such as fragmented systems, interoperability issues, and resistance to change. By serving as platforms for collaboration, Labs such as Mayo Clinic's Center for Innovation support healthcare organizations in navigating regulatory complexities, fostering a culture of innovation, and addressing technological and cultural barriers. These Labs also emphasize user-centered design and stakeholder engagement to ensure that the solutions developed are both effective and adaptable to real-world settings (Davenport and Bean, 2022).

Additionally, Innovation Labs leverage emerging technologies such as AI, IoT, and telemedicine to drive transformation. The Singapore General Hospital Innovation Lab, for example, integrates AI into workflows to enhance diagnostic precision and operational efficiency (Singapore General Hospital, 2024). These technologies not only improve patient experiences but also enable the development of new business models that address systemic inefficiencies and expand access to care. The Labs' ability to facilitate interdisciplinary collaboration and iterative development processes positions them as pivotal enablers of healthcare DT.

By addressing pressing healthcare challenges, Healthcare Innovation Labs demonstrate their capacity to act as catalysts for change.

Their emphasis on community-driven innovation, the facilitation of interdisciplinary partnerships, and the creation of scalable solutions underscores their strategic importance in the sector. As illustrated by the diverse case examples, these Labs provide robust frameworks for advancing healthcare DT and responding to the unique needs of the sector. This general understanding sets the stage for a deeper exploration of specific applications and real-world impacts of Innovation Labs in healthcare, showcasing how they overcome sector-specific challenges and contribute to digital health advancements.

5. Discussion: Leveraging Innovation Labs for Healthcare Transformation

The Innovation Lab highlights the enormous potential to promote DT in healthcare by tackling interesting challenges and promoting innovations that meet the evolving needs of patients, users, providers, and stakeholders. These laboratories serve as open platforms for collaboration, experimentation, and capacity building. Helping various organizations Able to navigate the complexities of DT, the following describes the diverse role of innovation labs in healthcare across five strategic dimensions: catalyzing digital transformation, promoting collaboration, fostering sustainable innovation, integrating equity and inclusivity, and promoting knowledge in digital innovation.

Catalyzing digital transformation in healthcare: Innovation Labs contribute to catalyzing DT within a structured environment where organizations are free to experiment with emerging technologies, such as AI, IoT, and telemedicine. In this vein, Labs work as testbeds and islands of experimentation. For example, the Finnish HealthHub hosts startups and established healthcare organizations to test digital solutions in controlled environment, guaranteeing rigorous validation without disrupting clinical workflows. These Labs support iterative development, enabling solutions to be refined based on real-world feedback. This approach not only mitigates the risk of failure but also accelerates the adoption of digital tools, thereby fostering a proactive and innovative healthcare culture. Moreover, the Labs contribute to the humanization of care by focusing on innovations that enhance the patient experience. Personalized health monitoring tools and patient-centric service platforms, often developed and validated within these Labs, empower patients to actively participate in their care journeys.

Promoting collaboration: The collaborative nature of Innovation Labs positions them as open innovation platforms that foster relationship building between diverse stakeholders. They stimulate the creation of opportunities for clinicians, researchers, startups, and policymakers, to co-create solutions tailored to real-world challenges. By facilitating such collaborations, these Labs enable skills and knowledge exchange, as well as resource sharing. This aspect is critical for addressing the above-discussed systemic healthcare challenges, such as interoperability and fragmented information systems. In this perspective, the role of these Labs is more than mere facilitation. They act as broker and mediators to align stakeholder interests, streamline communication, and foster the creation of a common shared pathway for innovation. This approach enhances the efficiency while controlling the risk of failure of innovation projects. So, it ensures that the projects are not only technically feasible but also socially and economically viable as well as tailored to the real needs perceived by the final recipients.

Fostering sustainable innovation: Sustainability is a cornerstone of effective healthcare innovation. Innovation Labs' approach strongly contribute in this sense. Lean and agile principles distinguishing Innovation Labs' management model allow Labs to manage projects in an adaptive manner, integrating diverse perspectives and responding to emerging challenges. In addition to sustainability in innovation, Labs foster resilience within healthcare organizations by creating adaptive pathways for change. Often, as in the case of the. Lecco Living Lab (Marone *et al.*, 2020), they provide training programs that equip healthcare professionals with the skills needed to navigate the complexities of DT. This adaptability is critical in a sector as dynamic and unpredictable as healthcare.

Integrating equity and inclusivity: Innovation Labs' approach is also aimed at addressing disparities in healthcare by promoting equity and inclusivity in their initiatives. By involving patients from diverse demographics in co-creation processes, Labs ensure that solutions serve heterogeneous needs, so as to reduce healthcare inequities. The Digital Health Living Lab at the University of Brighton (Fotis *et al.*, 2023), for instance, addresses this challenge, by involving surrounding communities in co-creation activities for the development of healthcare innovative solutions. Moreover, Healthcare Innovation Labs can also pursue more democratizing and ethical goals, in terms of, for example, developing cost-effective solutions that make advanced care accessible to under-served populations. Their emphasis on inclusivity, thus, ensures that the benefits of innovation are equitably distributed.

Promoting knowledge in digital innovation: Another critical barrier to healthcare DT is the digital divide and the lack of digital skills. Innovation Labs address this challenge by delivering training programs and/or workshops both for healthcare professionals and patients. Labs such as HealthHub Finland organize these kinds of workshops and training sessions to enhance digital skills, ensuring that recipients can effectively exploit the full potential of healthcare digital tools. By promoting educational initiatives, Labs ensure to break the silos where often innovation units reside. In this way, healthcare innovations are not only developed but also understood by the rest of the organization and adopted by intended users.

6. Conclusions: The Strategic Role of Innovation Labs in Healthcare Transformation

This research set out to explore and shed light on the emerging phenomenon of Innovation Labs in healthcare – a promising yet still underutilized approach in the sector. Through a combination of case examples and a comprehensive review of the literature, it has been possible to examine the potential of these Labs to address the persistent barriers to DT in healthcare. The findings reveal that Healthcare Innovation Labs prove to be an innovative emerging approach useful to overcoming challenges and unlocking opportunities in DT. Their multifaceted roles as testbeds, open platforms for collaboration, and catalysts for human-centered innovation highlight their potential to address systemic issues and drive digital transformative change. Being sure to align their activities with the strategic value proposition of healthcare organizations, these Labs ensure that innovative solutions are developed according to real needs so as to increase efficiency and enable effective implementation into healthcare systems.

Future studies could delve deeper into the case examples presented, transforming them into detailed case studies aimed at constructing theoretical frameworks for the management and functioning of healthcare Innovation Labs. These efforts would not only contribute to academic discourse but also provide practical insights for policymakers and practitioners. Such frameworks could guide the formulation of targeted policies and actionable strategies, ultimately facilitating the broader adoption and diffusion of Innovation Labs across the healthcare ecosystem. By doing so, these Labs can fulfill their potential as catalysts for sustainable, inclusive, and impactful innovation.

References

Agarwal, R., Gao, G., DesRoches, C., and Jha, A. K. (2010). Research commentary – The digital transformation of healthcare: Current status and the road ahead. *Information systems research, 21*(4), 796–809.

Al-haimi, B., Hujainah, F., Nasir, D., and Alhroob, E. (2021). Higher education institutions with artificial intelligence: Roles, promises, and requirements. In: Hamdan, A., Hassanien, A.E., Khamis, R., Alareeni, B., Razzaque, A., Awwad, B. (eds.), *Applications of Artificial Intelligence in Business, Education and Healthcare*, Vol. 954, Studies in Computational Intelligence. Springer, Cham.

Dash, S. P. (2020). The impact of IoT in healthcare: Global technological change & the roadmap to a networked architecture in India. *Journal of the Indian Institute of Science, 100*(4), 773–785.

Davenport, T. and Bean, R. (2022). AI-based innovations at mayo clinic. In MIT Sloan Management Review. Available at: https://sloanreview.mit.edu/article/ai-based-innovations-at-mayo-clinic.

De Silva, M. and Wright, M. (2019). Entrepreneurial co-creation: Societal impact through open innovation. *R&D Management, 49*(7), 12362.

Fecher, F., Winding, J., Hutter, K., and Füller, J. (2018). Innovation labs from a participants' perspective. *Journal of Business Research, 110*, 567–576.

Fotis, T., Kioskli, K., Sundaralingam, A., Fasihi, A., and Mouratidis, H. (2023). Co-creation in a digital health living lab: A case study. *Frontiers in Public Health, 10*, 892930.

Frisinger, A. and Papachristou, P. (2024). Bridging the voice of healthcare to digital transformation in practice – a holistic approach. *BMC Digital Health, 2*(1), 12.

Gopal, G., Suter-Crazzolara, C., Toldo, L., and Eberhardt, W. (2019). Digital transformation in healthcare – architectures of present and future information technologies. *Clinical Chemistry and Laboratory Medicine (CCLM), 57*(3), 328–335.

Healthcare Living Lab Catalonia (2024). Available at: https://healthcarelivinglab.cat/ (accessed November 12, 2024).

Hermes, S., Riasanow, T., Clemons, E. K., Böhm, M., and Krcmar, H. (2020). The digital transformation of the healthcare industry: exploring the rise of emerging platform ecosystems and their influence on the role of patients. *Business Research, 13*(3), 1033–1069.

Innovations in International Health (2024). Available at: https://web.archive.org/web/20100922214538/http://iih.mit.edu/ (accessed November 20, 2024).

Kakale, M. A. M. (2024). Of digital transformation in the healthcare (systematic review of the current state of the literature). *Health and Technology, 14*(1), 35–50.

Kane, G. C., Nanda, R., Phillips, A. N., and Copulsky, J. R. (2021). *The Transformation Myth: Leading Your Organization Through Uncertain Times.* MIT Press.

Khodadad-Saryazdi, A. (2021). Exploring the telemedicine implementation challenges through the process innovation approach: A case study research in the French healthcare sector. *Technovation, 107*, 102273.

Kraus, S., Schiavone, F., Pluzhnikova, A., and Invernizzi, A. C. (2021). Digital transformation in healthcare: Analysing the current state-of-research. *Journal of Business Research, 123*, 557–567.

Laurenza, E., Quintano, M., Schiavone, F., and Vrontis, D. (2018). The effect of digital technologies adoption in healthcare industry: A case based analysis. *Business Process Management Journal, 24*(5), 0084.

Lewis, M. and Moultrie, J. (2005). The organisational innovation laboratory. *Creativity and Innovation Management, 14*(1), 73–83.

Magadley, W. and Birdi, K. (2009). Innovation labs: An examination into the use of physical spaces to enhance organisational creativity. *Creativity and innovation management, 18*(4), 315–325.

Marone, L., Onofrio, R., and Masella, C. (2020). The Italian Case of Lecco Innovation Living Lab: Stakeholders' needs and activities to contribute to the technological innovation process in healthcare. *Sustainability, 12*(24), 10266.

Memon, A. B., Meyer, K., Thieme, M., and Meyer, L. P. (2018). Inter-InnoLab collaboration: An investigation of the diversity and interconnection among Innovation Laboratories. *Journal of Engineering and Technology Management, 47*, 1–21.

Meyer, M., Kuusisto, J., Grant, K., De Silva, M., Flowers, S., and Choksy, U. (2018). Towards new Triple Helix organisations? A comparative study of competence centres as knowledge, consensus and innovation spaces. *R&D Management, 49*(4), 555–573.

Molloy, S. (2018). *Innovation Labs in Healthcare: A Review of Design Labs as a Model for Healthcare Innovation.* Ocad University – Toronto, Ontario, Canada.

Morel, S., Unger, L., and Buet, G. (2016). Behind-the-scenes of eco-innovation at Renault: From collective action to breakthrough concepts. *International*

Journal on Interactive Design and Manufacturing (IJIDeM), *10*(3), 251–255.

Nambisan, S. (2017). Digital entrepreneurship: Toward a digital technology perspective of entrepreneurship. *Entrepreneurship Theory and Practice*, *41*(6), 1029–1055.

Osorio, F., Dupont, L., Camargo, M., Palominos, P., Peña, J. I., and Alfaro, M. (2019). Design and management of innovation laboratories: Toward a performance assessment tool. *Creativity and Innovation Management*, *28*(1), 82–100.

Peek, N., Sujan, M., and Scott, P. (2023). Digital health and care: Emerging from pandemic times. BMJ Health & Care Informatics, *30*(1), e100861.

Raimo, N., De Turi, I., Albergo, F., and Vitolla, F. (2022). The drivers of the digital transformation in the healthcare industry: An empirical analysis in Italian hospitals. *Technovation*, 102558.

Ravi, B. (2020). Medical device innovation: Idea to impact. In *Centenary Book "Engineering for the Future"*, pp. 371–383. Institution of Engineers (India).

Santarsiero, F., Schiuma, G., Carlucci, D., and Helander, N. (2023). Digital transformation in healthcare organisations: The role of innovation labs. *Technovation*, *122*, 102640.

Santarsiero, F., Carlucci, D., and Schiuma, G. (2024). Driving digital transformation and business model innovation in tourism through innovation labs: An empirical study. *Journal of Engineering and Technology Management*, *74*, 101841.

Scarmoncin, A., Portelli, C., Osorio, F., and Eckerlein, G. (2022). Unfolding innovation lab services in public hospitals: A hospital FabLab case study. In *2022 IEEE 28th International Conference on Engineering, Technology and Innovation (ICE/ITMC) & 31st International Association for Management of Technology (IAMOT) Joint Conference*, pp. 1–10. IEEE.

Schiuma, G. and Santarsiero, F. (2023). Innovation labs as organisational catalysts for innovation capacity development: A systematic literature review. *Technovation*, *123*, 102690.

Schiuma, G., Schettini, E., and Santarsiero, F. (2021). How wise companies drive digital transformation. *Journal of Open Innovation: Technology, Market, and Complexity*, *7*(2), 122.

Singapore General Hospital (2024). AI Lab. Available at: https://www.sgh.com.sg/Diagnostic-Radiology/Pages/Research/AI-Lab.aspx.

Sousa, M. J., Pesqueira, A., Lemos, C., Sousa, M., and Rocha, A. (2019). Decision-making based on big data analytics for people management in healthcare organizations. *Journal of Medical Systems*, *43*(9), 290.

Shaw, J., Abejirinde, I. O. O., Agarwal, P., Shahid, S., and Martin, D. (2024). Digital health and equitable access to care. *PLOS Digital Health*, *3*(9), e0000573.

Tasca, R., Ventura, I. L. S., Borges, V., Leles, F. A. G., Gomes, R. D. M., Ribas, A. N., Carvalho, W. M., and Jimenez, J. M. S. (2019). Health innovation laboratories: Towards strong primary health care (PHC) in the federal district of brasilia. *Ciência & Saúde Coletiva*, *24*, 2021–2030.

The Straits Times (2023). New AI tool helps SGH doctors predict risk of complications after surgery, May 3. Available at: https://www.straitstimes.com/singapore/new-ai-tool-helps-sgh-doctors-predict-risk-of-complications-after-surgery.

Tõnurist, P., Kattel, R., and Lember, V. (2017). Innovation labs in the public sector: what they are and what they do? *Public Management Review*, *19*(10), 1455–1479.

Tolomiczenko, G. and Sanger, T. (2015). Linking Engineering and Medical Training: A USC program seeks to introduce medical and engineering students to medical device development. *IEEE Pulse*, *6*(6), 32–36.

Torvinen, H. and Jansson, K. (2022). Public health care innovation lab tackling the barriers of public sector innovation. *Public Management Review*, 1–23.

Tucker, R. (2017). Starting an innovation lab? Avoid these pitfalls, 20 November. *Forbes*.

Chapter 3

Transforming and Democratizing Clinical Workflows: The Role of Large Language Models (LLMs) in Disrupting Healthcare

David M. Liebovitz

*Northwestern University Feinberg School of Medicine,
Chicago, IL, USA*

1. Introduction

Clinical workflows form the backbone of modern healthcare, yet they are increasingly overwhelmed by the dual pressures of growing administrative complexity and rising patient expectations. Physicians and nurses frequently report spending more time navigating electronic health records (EHRs) and tackling bureaucratic hurdles than engaging in direct patient care. This imbalance not only contributes to professional burnout but also diminishes the quality of care patients receive, eroding trust and satisfaction on both sides of the healthcare relationship.

The current state of clinical workflows presents significant challenges. Overloaded systems lead to fragmented communication, delayed care, and inefficient resource allocation. These inefficiencies undermine patient outcomes, intensify healthcare disparities, and perpetuate dissatisfaction across all stakeholders. Meanwhile, the administrative burden has reached unsustainable levels, with clinicians spending nearly twice as much time on documentation as on patient interaction (Sinsky *et al.*, 2016).

Amid these challenges, large language models (LLMs) – advanced artificial intelligence (AI) systems designed to process and generate human-like text – have emerged as transformative tools in healthcare. By automating routine documentation, facilitating communication, and delivering actionable insights, LLMs hold the potential to reshape clinical workflows. They can help clinicians refocus on what matters most: providing empathetic, high-quality care. For patients, these technologies promise personalized experiences, faster access to services, and improved health outcomes.

This chapter explores the role of LLMs in modernizing and democratizing healthcare. Beginning with an analysis of current pain points in clinical workflows, we examine how these technologies can address systemic inefficiencies and bridge the gap between providers and patients. By illustrating real-world applications and ethical considerations, we aim to envision a future where AI complements human expertise, enhancing both operational efficiency and the patient experience.

2. Current State of Clinical Workflows: Pain Points from the Clinician Perspective

In today's healthcare environment, clinicians face significant obstacles that hinder their ability to deliver optimal care. Overwhelming administrative demands, outdated communication systems, and time constraints dominate their workdays, detracting from patient care and contributing to burnout. These pain points highlight systemic inefficiencies that demand urgent attention.

2.1. *Administrative overload: The silent epidemic*

Healthcare providers often find themselves consumed by administrative tasks, leaving limited time for patient interactions. Consider a general practitioner managing a panel of 2,000 patients, many with chronic or complex conditions, such as congestive heart failure or cancer. Each case requires meticulous documentation, coordination of medications, diagnostic tests, and specialist referrals – tasks that create an unsustainable cognitive load.

EHRs, designed to streamline care, frequently exacerbate the problem. Providers spend hours navigating through verbose, unstructured documentation to extract critical information, often encountering redundant or missing data. For example, the widespread use of "copy-and-paste" functions can propagate errors and obscure crucial updates in a patient's record (Wrenn *et al.*, 2010).

Beyond documentation, patient portals – intended to facilitate communication – often add to clinicians' workloads. Answering non-urgent patient messages, reviewing records, and addressing follow-up questions can consume hours, yet this work is rarely compensated. The labyrinthine process of prior authorizations further compounds the issue. Clinicians must spend precious time negotiating with insurers, delaying necessary diagnostics or treatments, and frustrating both patients and providers.

The cumulative effect of these demands is profound. Administrative overload disrupts clinical reasoning, reduces job satisfaction, and is a major contributor to physician burnout, with some studies reporting burnout rates exceeding well over 50% among healthcare providers (Rotenstein, 2018).

2.2. *Outdated communication systems: Fragmentation and inefficiency*

Despite advancements in technology, healthcare communication remains archaic in many respects. Fax machines – a relic of the past – persist as standard tools in clinical settings, leading to delays, misplaced documents, and inefficiencies.

Interoperability, or the seamless exchange of information across different systems, remains another significant challenge. Providers frequently must synthesize fragmented patient data from disparate EHR systems, laboratory databases, and imaging platforms. This lack of cohesive communication hinders timely decision-making, increases the risk of errors, and perpetuates redundant testing.

Moreover, communication within care teams is often suboptimal. Busy clinicians may struggle to coordinate across departments, creating bottlenecks in workflows. Inadequate communication infrastructure not only affects operational efficiency but also compromises patient safety and satisfaction.

2.3. *Time constraints: A race against the clock*

The growing complexity of healthcare and the increasing demand for services have created relentless time pressures for clinicians. Many providers must navigate packed schedules, leaving little room to fully address patients' concerns. For example, a primary care physician typically has 15–20 minutes per appointment – time that must cover history-taking, physical examination, charting, and care planning.

This scarcity of time forces clinicians to prioritize efficiency over depth, often at the expense of meaningful patient–provider interactions. Patients may leave visits feeling unheard, while providers grapple with the frustration of insufficient time to address all aspects of care. This transactional nature of appointments undermines trust, satisfaction, and the overall quality of care.

2.4. *Bottlenecks in access to specialized care*

For patients requiring specialized care, the journey is often fraught with delays. Wait times for subspecialist appointments can stretch for weeks or months, leading to worsening conditions and increased anxiety. Clinicians, left without timely expert input, face the challenge of managing complex cases alone.

Emergency departments, which serve as a critical safety net, are similarly burdened. Long wait times discourage patients from seeking timely care and strain providers who must triage high volumes of cases. These delays reflect a healthcare system at its breaking point, unable to meet the needs of its most vulnerable patients.

2.5. *Conclusion*

The pain points outlined above paint a stark picture of the current state of clinical workflows. Administrative burdens, outdated communication systems, time constraints, and access bottlenecks are deeply entrenched challenges that compromise both provider well-being and patient outcomes. Addressing these issues requires transformative solutions – solutions that LLMs and AI-powered tools have the potential to deliver.

3. Current State of Healthcare Delivery: The Patient's Perspective

For patients, navigating the healthcare system often feels like navigating an intricate maze – overwhelming, inefficient, and laden with barriers. Despite advancements in technology and healthcare delivery, many patients continue to encounter communication breakdowns, system fragmentation, and limited access to timely care. These challenges not only hinder patient satisfaction but also exacerbate inequities and negatively impact health outcomes.

3.1. *Communication breakdowns: A barrier to clarity and connection*

Effective communication is essential for trust and collaboration between patients and providers. However, many patients find themselves frustrated by unanswered questions, delayed responses, and impersonal interactions.

Patient portals, while promising greater accessibility, often fall short in practice. Messages sent through these platforms can go unanswered for days or weeks, leaving patients anxious and uncertain (Children's Hospital Association, 2022). For example, a patient reporting a new symptom through a portal may receive an automated response instructing them to call the office – a solution that often leads to further delays. Similarly, trying to reach a provider by phone frequently involves navigating a web of automated menus or long hold times, compounding patient frustration.

Moreover, medical jargon and complex test results further alienate patients. A person managing chronic conditions, such as diabetes or heart disease, may feel overwhelmed by technical language that obscures actionable insights. For instance, a change in lab results may prompt anxiety: Is this dangerous? Does it require immediate attention? Without clear, timely guidance, patients are left to interpret critical information on their own, risking mismanagement of their condition.

3.2. *Fragmented systems: A maze of care coordination*

The healthcare system's fragmentation presents significant hurdles for patients, especially those with complex medical needs. Coordinating care among multiple specialists often feels like managing separate, unconnected teams, each with its own communication style, scheduling system, and patient portal.

Insurance-related challenges further complicate the patient experience. Processes such as prior authorization create frustrating delays, leaving patients unsure whether crucial diagnostics or treatments will be approved. For example, a cancer patient awaiting authorization for a follow-up scan may experience unnecessary anxiety and worsening health due to procedural delays.

This fragmentation often leads to gaps in care. Missed follow-ups, inconsistent advice from different providers, and redundant tests not only burden patients but also waste resources and increase the likelihood of medical errors.

3.3. *The time crunch: Limited provider access*

Short appointment durations often leave patients feeling rushed and unheard. With visits sometimes capped at 15 minutes, patients may struggle to articulate their concerns or ask meaningful questions. This lack of time also makes it difficult to explore holistic issues, such as the impact of lifestyle, mental health, or personal stressors on their medical conditions.

The time constraints don't end in the exam room. Patients seeking specialized care often face weeks- or months-long delays for appointments. These protracted wait times exacerbate medical conditions, create emotional distress, and widen disparities, particularly for underserved populations. Such delays often force patients to rely on emergency departments for conditions that could have been managed through timely outpatient care, placing further strain on an already overburdened system.

3.4. *Self-management: Empowerment or burden?*

Modern healthcare increasingly emphasizes patient self-management, where individuals take a more active role in monitoring their health and adhering to treatment plans. While this shift aims to empower patients, it often imposes significant burdens, particularly for those without adequate resources or support.

For example, a patient discharged after surgery may be instructed to monitor for signs of infection, manage pain medications, and schedule follow-up visits – all while dealing with other life demands, such as caregiving or financial stress. Without clear guidance or consistent follow-up, patients can feel overwhelmed and uncertain.

Patients are also expected to advocate for their own care, navigate insurance processes, request referrals, and ensure continuity among multiple providers. For individuals unfamiliar with the healthcare system or hesitant to assert their needs, this expectation can become a barrier to effective care.

3.5. *Case study: Lisa's struggle in a fragmented system*

Background: Lisa, a 52-year-old woman managing type 2 diabetes, hypertension, and sleep apnea, faces numerous challenges in navigating her care. Despite her proactive approach to managing her health through diet, exercise, and medication, systemic inefficiencies leave her frustrated and vulnerable.

Key challenges:
1. *Communication breakdowns*: Lisa's multiple providers use different patient portals, leading to confusion and missed updates on her care plan.
2. *Insurance hurdles*: Delayed prior authorization for a continuous glucose monitor (CGM) results in her blood sugar spiking and a subsequent emergency department visit.
3. *Time constraints*: Short appointment durations prevent Lisa from addressing all her concerns, resulting in miscommunications and gaps in her care.
4. *Fragmented records*: Lisa struggles to manage her medications, test results, and appointments with different specialists, leading to missed follow-ups and unnecessary stress.

Outcome: Lisa's experience highlights how communication failures, insurance delays, and fragmented care coordination create significant barriers to effective healthcare delivery. Despite her best efforts, systemic obstacles compromise her ability to manage her health effectively.

Relevant statistics:
Communication: While patient portals are becoming more common, their adoption remains limited, with only 31.4% of individuals using them in

2018 (National Cancer Institute, 2020). Disparities based on sex, income, and education levels further compound this issue. Despite these tools, many patients continue to rely on traditional methods such as phone calls for communication, though specific data quantifying this reliance remain limited (The Medical Care Blog, 2017).

Navigation: Insurance-related confusion and financial concerns frequently delay care. For example, in 2022, 8% of adults reported delaying or not receiving medical care due to cost (Health System Tracker, 2022). Additionally, disparities in patient portal use hinder effective care coordination among patients managing multiple providers (Yamin *et al.*, 2022).

Access: Time constraints and systemic inefficiencies continue to limit access to care. While specific data on primary care appointment durations and time allocated for patient questions remain elusive, delays in accessing specialist care are widely acknowledged. Systemic factors such as insurance approvals exacerbate these delays (U.S. News & World Report, 2023).

Self-management: Patients managing chronic conditions often rely on patient portals, with 70.5% engaging with these tools. However, disparities in portal use suggest that many patients still struggle to manage their health effectively between appointments (JAMA Network Open, 2023). Furthermore, many patients report feeling responsible for coordinating their own care, often without sufficient support (JAMA Network Open, 2023).

3.6. *Conclusion*

The challenges faced by patients such as Lisa reveal systemic inefficiencies that hinder their ability to access, navigate, and benefit from healthcare services. Fragmented communication, limited provider access, and an increasing reliance on self-management create unnecessary stress and inequity. Addressing these barriers is essential to improving the patient experience and ensuring equitable, high-quality care. As we explore the potential of LLMs in healthcare, their ability to simplify processes, enhance communication, and empower patients offers a pathway toward a more efficient and compassionate system.

References

- Health System Tracker (2022). How does cost affect access to care? Available at: https://www.healthsystemtracker.org/chart-collection/cost-affect-access-care (accessed December 14, 2024).
- JAMA Network Open (2023). Disparities in patient portal engagement among patients with hypertension. Available at: https://jamanetwork.com/journals/jamanetworkopen/fullarticle/2818725 (accessed December 14, 2024).
- National Cancer Institute (2020). Patient portals and online health information exchange: HINTS brief 45. Available at: https://hints.cancer.gov/docs/Briefs/HINTS_Brief_45.pdf (accessed December 14, 2024).
- The Medical Care Blog (2017). Patient portals, part 2: Barriers and challenges. Available at: https://www.themedicalcareblog.com/patient-portals-part-2 (accessed December 14, 2024).
- U.S. News & World Report (2023). Health insurance barriers delay, disrupt and deny patient care. Available at: https://www.usnews.com/opinion/articles/2023-08-08/health-insurance-barriers-delay-disrupt-and-deny-patient-care (accessed December 14, 2024).
- Yamin, C. K., Emani, S., Williams, D. H. *et al.* (2022). Patient portals and health information exchange. Journal of the American Medical Informatics Association. Available at: https://academic.oup.com/jamiaopen/article/5/4/ooac104/6887151 (accessed December 14, 2024).

4. The AI-Powered Clinic: LLMs Transforming Healthcare Delivery

The growing complexity of healthcare systems calls for innovative solutions to address inefficiencies, improve patient outcomes, and alleviate provider burnout. LLMs, such as OpenAI's GPT models, represent a significant step forward in AI, offering tools capable of revolutionizing healthcare delivery. By integrating LLMs into clinical workflows, organizations can streamline operations, enhance communication, and refocus care on patients.

4.1. *Automating documentation and administrative tasks*

Administrative responsibilities consume a significant portion of clinicians' time, contributing to inefficiency and burnout. LLMs offer solutions that streamline these tasks, enabling providers to dedicate more attention to patient care.

1. *AI-generated clinical documentation*: LLMs equipped with natural language processing (NLP) can transform the documentation process. Integrated with voice recognition technology, these systems can capture conversations during patient visits, extracting key information to generate accurate and comprehensive clinical notes. For example:
   * *Real-time documentation*: An AI assistant listens during consultations, automatically identifying symptoms, diagnoses, and treatment plans to populate EHRs without manual entry.
   * *Trend analysis*: LLMs can analyze historical patient data to highlight trends, such as declining kidney function or improving HbA1c levels, ensuring clinicians have a holistic view of patient health.

     This automation minimizes errors and reduces the cognitive load on providers, improving accuracy and allowing for more meaningful patient interactions.
2. *Enhancing patient portal interactions*: Patient portals are critical tools for communication but often overwhelm clinicians. LLMs can streamline portal workflows by
   * generating automated responses to routine questions (e.g., medication refills, appointment scheduling),
   * triaging urgent messages to ensure timely provider review,
   * providing natural language query support, enabling patients to ask questions such as "When was my last cholesterol test?" and receive clear, actionable answers.
3. *Simplifying insurance processes*: Navigating insurance systems is a major administrative hurdle. LLMs can assist by
   * pre-filling prior authorization forms using patient data from EHRs,

- automating insurance claim coding to improve accuracy and reduce rejections,
- identifying cost-effective treatment options or financial assistance programs for patients, reducing the financial burden.

4.2. *Enhancing communication and care coordination*

Effective communication and coordination are essential for high-quality care. LLMs address systemic challenges by facilitating seamless information exchange and improving care transitions.

1. *Bridging communication gaps*:
   - *Digitizing legacy systems*: LLMs can transform handwritten notes and faxed documents into searchable, structured records, reducing reliance on outdated technology.
   - *Overcoming language barriers*: Equipped with real-time translation capabilities, LLMs enable providers to communicate effectively with patients who speak different languages, fostering trust and improving outcomes.
   - *Secure messaging*: By integrating with HIPAA-compliant platforms, LLMs facilitate secure and efficient information sharing between providers and across healthcare organizations.
2. *Optimizing care transitions*: Care transitions, such as moving a patient from the emergency department to an inpatient unit, are particularly vulnerable to communication breakdowns. LLMs can
   - automatically generate handoff summaries, ensuring providers receive concise and accurate updates,
   - monitor patient data for critical changes, triggering alerts to ensure timely interventions,
   - streamline interdepartmental referrals and follow-up scheduling, reducing delays and improving continuity of care.

4.3. *Optimizing patient–provider interactions*

The patient–provider relationship lies at the heart of healthcare. LLMs enhance this dynamic by supporting clinical decision-making, improving engagement, and fostering collaboration.

1. *Augmenting clinical decision-making* LLMs can assist providers by
   - analyzing patient data in real time to offer diagnostic suggestions and treatment recommendations, particularly for complex or rare conditions,
   - highlighting relevant research and guidelines tailored to a patient's unique health profile, enabling evidence-based decision-making,
   - identifying potential risks, such as contraindications or early warning signs of complications, to support proactive interventions.
2. *Increasing patient engagement*:
   - *Automated reminders*: LLMs can send personalized reminders for appointments, screenings, and medication adherence, reducing missed visits and improving compliance.
   - *Personalized education*: By generating easy-to-understand resources tailored to a patient's condition, LLMs empower individuals to take an active role in managing their health.
   - *Convenient communication*: AI-powered chat tools provide patients with accessible channels to ask questions, express concerns, and receive prompt support, strengthening trust and collaboration.

4.4. *Improving access to timely care*

Timely care is essential for optimal outcomes, yet long wait times and system inefficiencies often delay treatment. LLMs address these challenges by streamlining access to services and improving resource allocation.

1. *Prioritizing referrals*:
   - *AI-driven triage*: LLMs analyze referral information to assess urgency, ensuring patients with critical needs are prioritized.
   - *Virtual consultations*: For non-urgent cases, virtual visits can pre-screen patients, reducing the need for in-person appointments and freeing up resources for those requiring face-to-face care.
2. *Optimizing emergency department (ED) flow*:
   - *AI-assisted triage*: LLMs can analyze patient data upon arrival to prioritize cases by severity, reducing wait times and ensuring timely interventions.
   - *Real-time monitoring*: AI systems track ED wait times, patient volume, and resource availability, enabling dynamic adjustments to workflows.

4.5. *Conclusion*

By addressing key inefficiencies in documentation, communication, and patient access, LLMs offer transformative potential for healthcare delivery. These technologies enable clinicians to reclaim time for direct patient care, foster meaningful interactions, and improve the overall patient experience. As we integrate LLMs into healthcare systems, their role as tools for operational efficiency and patient empowerment highlights a promising path toward a more effective and equitable healthcare ecosystem.

5. Democratizing Healthcare: Empowering Patients with AI Tools

The convergence of advanced AI technologies and patient-centered care is revolutionizing how individuals engage with their health. LLMs play a pivotal role in this transformation, empowering patients to manage their care, access critical information, and navigate complex systems with greater autonomy. By enhancing personalization, simplifying processes, and expanding access, LLMs contribute to a more inclusive and equitable healthcare system.

5.1. *AI-driven personalized guidance*

Personalized care is a necessity for effective healthcare delivery. LLMs enable tailored interventions that meet the unique needs of individual patients.

1. *Behavioral nudges for improved adherence*: Imagine receiving a timely, discreet reminder to take your medication, attend a follow-up appointment, or schedule a preventive screening. LLMs analyze a patient's health data to deliver personalized prompts, fostering adherence without being intrusive. These nudges can align with patients' preferences and routines, promoting engagement while reducing care gaps.

2. *Self-scheduling and preventive care*: LLMs can identify when patients are due for screenings, check-ups, or vaccinations based on their medical history. They facilitate self-scheduling through user-friendly interfaces, eliminating barriers such as phone call queues or complex

scheduling systems. For example, a patient managing hypertension might receive a message suggesting a follow-up visit, with the option to book an appointment in a few clicks.

5.2. *AI-facilitated second opinions and safety monitoring*

LLMs enhance patient safety by providing additional layers of oversight and proactive monitoring.

1. *Automated second opinions*: By analyzing medical records and clinical data, LLMs can generate preliminary second opinions, offering new insights or confirming existing treatment plans. For instance, an AI-driven review might identify alternative medication options for a patient experiencing adverse effects, ensuring care remains optimized.
2. *Continuous safety monitoring*: LLMs can actively monitor patient data, such as medication lists, lab results, and imaging reports, for potential safety concerns. These systems can
   - flag potential drug interactions or contraindications,
   - highlight abnormal lab trends that require immediate attention,
   - alert care teams to critical findings that may otherwise be overlooked (e.g., results from an outside ED visit), ensuring timely interventions.

5.3. *Enhancing patient advocacy and cost-effectiveness*

Navigating the complexities of healthcare systems can be daunting. LLMs empower patients to advocate for themselves more effectively while identifying cost-saving opportunities.

1. *Streamlining cost management*: AI tools can monitor prescription prices across pharmacies to find the most affordable options, helping patients save on medication costs. LLMs can also assist providers in selecting cost-effective treatments or applying for financial assistance programs. For example, a patient prescribed an expensive medication might receive suggestions for lower-cost alternatives or pharmaceutical discount programs.
2. *Simplifying health literacy*: Patients often struggle to understand medical jargon and complex care plans. LLMs can break down technical language into clear, actionable explanations, enabling patients to

make informed decisions. Whether clarifying test results or explaining treatment options, these tools foster confidence and autonomy in managing health.

5.4. *Expanding access to care*

LLMs bridge gaps in healthcare access, particularly for underserved populations, by enabling remote and virtual care solutions.

1. *AI-enhanced virtual assistants*: Patients in rural or resource-limited areas often face challenges accessing timely care. LLM-powered virtual assistants can provide the following:
   - *Remote monitoring*: Tracking chronic conditions such as diabetes through wearable devices, with AI tools offering insights and alerts for abnormal readings.
   - *On-demand guidance*: Answering basic health-related questions in real time, reducing unnecessary clinic visits while ensuring patients feel supported.
   - *Symptom checkers*: Guiding patients to appropriate care settings based on symptom severity, helping avoid overuse of emergency departments.
2. *Facilitating cross-language communication*: For patients facing language barriers, LLMs with translation capabilities offer an invaluable service. By bridging linguistic divides, these tools ensure patients can effectively communicate their concerns and understand medical advice, reducing disparities and improving care quality.

5.5. *Case study: Empowering patient engagement with AI*

Background: Mark, a 58-year-old patient with type 2 diabetes, faces challenges managing his condition, including medication adherence and understanding his lab results. Additionally, he struggles with rising prescription costs and lives in a rural area with limited access to specialists.

AI-driven solutions:
1. *Behavioral nudges*: Mark receives personalized reminders to take his medication and schedule follow-up appointments, improving adherence.

2. *Cost optimization*: An AI assistant identifies an affordable alternative to his prescribed insulin and connects him with a pharmaceutical savings program.
3. *Virtual care support*: Mark uses a virtual assistant to track his blood sugar levels and receives tailored insights, such as adjusting his diet to stabilize readings.
4. *Clear health guidance*: LLMs simplify his lab results, highlighting areas of concern and explaining the next steps in an accessible manner.

Outcome: With AI-powered support, Mark feels more in control of his health, reduces his healthcare costs, and avoids complications through improved adherence and proactive management.

5.6. Conclusion

By empowering patients with tools that enhance personalization, accessibility, and advocacy, LLMs democratize healthcare and foster a more patient-centered system. These technologies provide timely guidance, improve safety, and expand access to care for underserved populations. As healthcare increasingly shifts toward proactive and preventive models, the integration of LLMs offers a pathway to greater equity, efficiency, and empowerment.

6. Ethical, Regulatory, and Operational Challenges

While LLMs hold immense potential to revolutionize healthcare, their adoption also raises significant ethical, regulatory, and operational challenges. Addressing these concerns is critical to ensuring that these technologies are implemented responsibly, equitably, and effectively.

6.1. Ensuring accuracy and reliability

The accuracy of LLM outputs is paramount in healthcare, where decisions based on incorrect information can have dire consequences.

1. *Potential for errors*: LLMs are only as reliable as the data on which they are trained. Biases in training datasets or limitations in

domain-specific knowledge can lead to inaccurate recommendations or outputs. For instance:

- *Incomplete data contexts*: LLMs may provide recommendations based on partial patient histories, overlooking critical nuances.
- *Overconfidence in outputs*: The tendency of LLMs to generate plausible-sounding but incorrect responses ("hallucinations") poses risks in medical applications.

2. *Mitigation strategies*:
   - *Human oversight*: All AI-generated outputs should undergo review by qualified healthcare professionals, particularly in high-risk contexts, such as diagnostics and treatment planning.
   - *Error monitoring and feedback*: Continuous auditing of LLM performance, along with mechanisms for error reporting, ensures iterative improvements.
   - *Validation protocols*: Using multiple AI systems to cross-check outputs or integrating LLMs with domain-specific knowledge bases can enhance reliability.

6.2. *Protecting data privacy and security*

Healthcare data is among the most sensitive information, and its protection is a legal, ethical, and operational imperative.

1. *Regulatory compliance*: LLMs must adhere to stringent privacy standards, including the Health Insurance Portability and Accountability Act (HIPAA) in the United States and General Data Protection Regulation (GDPR) in Europe. Ensuring compliance involves the following:
   - *Data encryption*: Securing data at rest and during transmission to prevent unauthorized access.
   - *Access controls*: Restricting user permissions to minimize the risk of breaches.
2. *Mitigating third-party risks*: Many healthcare AI tools rely on third-party vendors. Organizations must
   - conduct thorough risk assessments, including vendor audits and penetration testing,
   - require contractual guarantees regarding data use, storage, and disposal.

3. *Anonymization and de-identification*: To enable safe data sharing for AI training or analytics, robust de-identification protocols must be implemented. These processes should strike a balance between preserving data utility and protecting patient identities.

6.3. Navigating regulatory challenges

The integration of LLMs into healthcare must align with evolving regulatory frameworks, which vary across jurisdictions and applications.

1. *Approval processes*: AI tools used in clinical decision-making may require regulatory approval, such as from the U.S. Food and Drug Administration (FDA). To streamline this process,
    *   developers should engage with regulatory agencies early in the design phase,
    *   robust documentation of training, validation, and testing should be maintained to demonstrate safety and efficacy.
2. *Patient-initiated actions*: LLMs enabling patient autonomy, such as self-scheduling advanced tests, may introduce new regulatory complexities. Clear guidelines must address liability and safety concerns while supporting patient empowerment.

6.4. Addressing equity and access

AI in healthcare must be implemented in ways that reduce, rather than exacerbate, disparities in care.

1. *Bridging the digital divide*: The cost of developing and deploying LLMs may create barriers for under-resourced healthcare systems. Strategies to promote equitable access include
    *   public–private partnerships to subsidize AI integration in underserved areas,
    *   open-source AI platforms designed to be accessible and affordable.
2. *Inclusive design*: LLMs must be trained on diverse datasets to reflect the needs of different populations. Additionally,
    *   models should account for linguistic diversity, ensuring accessibility for non-English speakers.

- feedback loops should be established to monitor and address potential disparities in outcomes. Unless carefully monitored and adjusted, algorithms may have differential effects on population segments (Obermeyer *et al.*, 2019).

6.5. *Ensuring transparency and building trust*

LLMs must be designed and deployed in ways that foster trust among patients, providers, and stakeholders.

1. *Explainability and interpretability*: Black-box AI systems, where decision-making processes are opaque, can erode trust. To enhance transparency,
   - models should generate explanations for their outputs in clear, non-technical language,
   - efforts to make AI processes interpretable for clinicians can facilitate informed decision-making.
2. *Open communication*: Healthcare organizations must proactively communicate AI capabilities, limitations, and safeguards to patients and providers. Educational initiatives, such as training modules for clinicians, can demystify LLM technology and promote confidence in its use.

6.6. *Addressing bias and discrimination*

Bias in AI systems can perpetuate or exacerbate healthcare inequities if not addressed.

1. *Sources of bias*:
   - Training data that underrepresents certain demographic groups can lead to disparities in recommendations or outcomes.
   - Pre-existing biases in healthcare, such as unequal access to care, may be reflected or amplified in AI outputs.
2. Strategies for mitigation:
   - *Diverse data inclusion*: Incorporating diverse, representative datasets in training and testing phases.
   - *Bias audits*: Regularly evaluating model performance across demographic groups to identify and address disparities.

- *Feedback mechanisms*: Allowing users to report biased outputs for continuous model improvement.

6.7. *Maintaining the human touch in healthcare*

While LLMs enhance efficiency, their integration must preserve the empathetic, human-centered aspects of care.

1. *Balancing efficiency and empathy*: AI should reduce administrative burdens, allowing clinicians more time for direct patient interactions. Training programs can emphasize the importance of maintaining a compassionate bedside manner, even in AI-augmented environments.
2. *Ethical frameworks*: Healthcare organizations should adopt ethical guidelines that prioritize patient well-being, informed consent, and respect for autonomy. These frameworks should guide the use of LLMs to enhance, rather than replace, the human elements of care.

6.8. *Conclusion*

The transformative potential of LLMs in healthcare is matched by the complexity of the ethical, regulatory, and operational challenges they present. Addressing these issues requires a multidisciplinary approach involving policymakers, technologists, and healthcare providers. By prioritizing accuracy, privacy, equity, and trust, organizations can harness LLMs to create a healthcare system that is both innovative and patient-centered.

7. The Future of Clinical Workflows and Patient-Led Disruption with LLMs

As healthcare continues to evolve, LLMs are poised to transform clinical workflows and empower patients in unprecedented ways. Moving beyond current applications, future integrations of LLMs will prioritize personalized care, predictive analytics, and proactive health management. These advancements will not only enhance the efficiency of healthcare delivery but also redefine the roles of providers and patients, creating a more collaborative, patient-led model of care.

7.1. Fully integrated and AI-enhanced systems

Healthcare's future lies in seamless integration, where LLMs act as central hubs, connecting disparate data sources and streamlining workflows.

1. *Unified data ecosystems*: The next generation of LLMs will enable real-time integration of patient data across platforms, such as EHRs, wearable devices, and laboratory systems. This unified ecosystem will
   - provide clinicians with a comprehensive, up-to-date patient profile to inform decision-making,
   - empower patients with simplified access to their own health data, enabling them to actively participate in their care.
2. *Enhanced efficiency for providers*: LLMs will eliminate many of the administrative redundancies that currently hinder workflows. Tasks such as prior authorizations, referral coordination, and insurance claims processing will become fully automated, allowing providers to focus on clinical care. By reducing administrative time, these systems will improve job satisfaction and alleviate burnout among healthcare professionals.

7.2. Predictive analytics and preventive care

As LLMs become more advanced, their ability to leverage large datasets for predictive insights will revolutionize healthcare's focus, shifting it from reactive treatment to proactive prevention.

1. *Early detection of health risks*: Through the analysis of patient records, biometrics, and even social determinants of health, LLMs will predict individual risk factors for chronic diseases, such as diabetes, heart disease, and cancer. These predictive models will
   - enable early interventions, improving outcomes and reducing costs,
   - provide tailored recommendations for lifestyle changes or preventive screenings.
2. *Population health management*: LLMs will play a crucial role in addressing public health challenges by analyzing trends across large populations. For example,
   - identifying communities at risk for outbreaks or chronic disease clusters,

- tailoring interventions (including visit scheduling) to address specific health inequities based on demographic, geographic, or socioeconomic data.

7.3. *From augmentation to transformation*

While LLMs currently augment provider workflows, their future potential lies in fundamentally transforming care delivery systems.

1. *Dynamic decision-making*: Future LLMs will serve as real-time collaborators for clinicians, synthesizing vast amounts of data to support complex clinical decisions. For example:
   - A physician treating a patient with multiple chronic conditions will receive evidence-based recommendations that consider all aspects of the patient's medical history, current condition, and social context.
   - In emergencies, LLMs could rapidly analyze incoming data to prioritize interventions, ensuring that care is both timely and precise.
2. *Empowered patients*: LLMs will provide patients with tools to take greater control of their healthcare. Personalized apps powered by AI will enable
   - continuous monitoring and management of chronic conditions,
   - accessible explanations of medical information, empowering patients to make informed decisions and advocate for their needs.

7.4. *The rise of patient-initiated care*

The integration of LLMs will shift healthcare from a provider-dominated model to one where patients actively lead their care journeys.

1. *Proactive health management*: Patients will use AI-powered platforms to monitor their health, identify potential risks, and access resources without waiting for provider intervention. For instance:
   - A patient experiencing new symptoms might use an LLM-powered virtual assistant to determine whether immediate medical attention is necessary or if self-care measures are sufficient.

- Self-scheduling tools will recommend appropriate appointments or screenings based on individual health profiles and medical histories.
2. *Addressing disparities in access*: LLMs will help bridge gaps in healthcare access, particularly in underserved regions. Virtual consultations, remote monitoring, and AI-driven health education tools will provide patients in rural or low-resource areas with access to high-quality care and expertise.

7.5. *Ethical and human-centered innovations*

As healthcare becomes increasingly digital, it will be essential to balance technological advancements with ethical considerations and human connection.

1. *Maintaining equity*: To ensure equitable access to LLM-enabled care, developers and policymakers must prioritize inclusivity. This includes designing systems that
   - accommodate diverse languages and literacy levels,
   - address cultural and socioeconomic barriers to AI adoption.
2. *Human oversight and empathy*: While LLMs will enhance efficiency, the human touch in healthcare must remain central. Providers will need to balance AI tools with empathetic communication, using the time saved through automation to strengthen patient relationships.

7.6. *Conclusion*

The future of clinical workflows and patient care with LLMs promises a paradigm shift toward efficiency, personalization, and equity. By fully integrating AI-powered tools into healthcare systems, providers can deliver proactive, patient-centered care that addresses both individual and population-level needs. For patients, the rise of accessible, AI-driven tools will enable greater autonomy, improved outcomes, and a more inclusive healthcare experience.

As LLMs continue to advance, thoughtful implementation will be crucial to ensuring that these technologies enhance – not replace – the human elements of care. By embracing this transformative potential responsibly, the healthcare ecosystem can create a future that is truly collaborative, compassionate, and innovative.

8. Conclusion

Healthcare today faces critical challenges, from administrative inefficiencies and fragmented workflows to inequitable access and overburdened providers. These systemic issues not only compromise the quality of care but also diminish patient satisfaction and exacerbate disparities. LLMs represent a transformative opportunity to address these challenges and reimagine healthcare delivery.

Through automation, predictive insights, and enhanced communication, LLMs can streamline clinical workflows, empower providers, and personalize patient care. By reducing administrative burdens, LLMs free clinicians to focus on building meaningful connections with patients. For individuals navigating the complexities of the healthcare system, these technologies provide tailored guidance, accessible information, and tools to actively manage their health.

However, the adoption of LLMs comes with significant ethical, regulatory, and operational considerations. Ensuring accuracy, protecting data privacy, addressing bias, and maintaining transparency are critical to building trust in these technologies. Moreover, the human touch must remain central to healthcare. LLMs should enhance – not replace – the empathetic interactions that form the foundation of patient-centered care.

Looking ahead, the integration of LLMs into healthcare systems holds immense potential to create a more equitable, efficient, and patient-driven ecosystem. By prioritizing inclusivity and responsible implementation, healthcare leaders can harness AI to improve outcomes, reduce disparities, and foster collaboration between providers and patients.

The path forward will require thoughtful innovation, cross-disciplinary collaboration, and a steadfast commitment to patient well-being. If embraced with care, LLMs can be powerful tools to bridge the gaps in modern healthcare and shape a future that is both technologically advanced and deeply compassionate.

Appendix: Resources for Further Exploration

To further deepen your understanding of LLMs and their applications in healthcare, we have compiled a list of valuable resources:

Interactive tools and experiments:
- *LLM Colab notebook*: This Google Colab notebook allows you to download and run a small language model, providing a hands-on experience with LLM technology.
  - https://bit.ly/llm-colab.

Podcasts and educational content:
- *Attention is All You Need – Podcast*: This AI-generated podcast delves into the foundational Google paper, "Attention is All You Need," and explores its connection to modern LLMs, such as ChatGPT and Google Gemini.
  - https://bit.ly/llm-attention.

Further Reading

General overviews of AI and LLMs in Healthcare

1. Topol, E. J. (2019). *Deep Medicine: How Artificial Intelligence Can Make Healthcare Human Again.* Basic Books.
   - This book provides a comprehensive exploration of how AI technologies, including natural language processing, can transform healthcare workflows and improve patient care.
2. Beam, A. L. and Kohane, I. S. (2018). Big data and machine learning in health care. *JAMA, 319*(13), 1317–1318. https://doi.org/10.1001/jama.2017.18391.
   - Discusses the potential of big data and machine learning, including LLMs, to address inefficiencies in clinical workflows and improve health outcomes.
3. Esteva, A., Robicquet, A., Ramsundar, B., Kuleshov, V., DePristo, M., Chou, K., Cui, C., Corrado, G., Thrun, S., and Dean, J. (2019). A guide to deep learning in healthcare. *Nature Medicine, 25*(1), 24–29. https://doi.org/10.1038/s41591-018-0316-z.
   - Highlights the applications of AI, particularly deep learning, in transforming healthcare, including workflow optimization.

Current challenges in clinical workflows

4. Children's Hospital Association (2022). How to improve portal messaging workflow. *Children's Hospitals Today.* Available at: https://www.childrenshospitals.org/news/childrens-hospitals-today/2022/07/how-to-improve-portal-messaging-workflow.

- Messages sent through these platforms can go unanswered for days or weeks, leaving patients anxious and uncertain.

5. Shanafelt, T. D. and Noseworthy, J. H. (2017). Executive leadership and physician well-being: Nine organizational strategies to promote engagement and reduce burnout. *Mayo Clinic Proceedings, 92*(1), 129–146. https://doi.org/10.1016/j.mayocp.2016.10.004.
    - Examines how workflow inefficiencies contribute to burnout and how systemic solutions could improve engagement and productivity.

6. Sinsky, C., Colligan, L., Li, L., Prgomet, M., Reynolds, S., Goeders, L., Westbrook, J., Tutty, M., and Blike, G. (2016). Allocation of physician time in ambulatory practice: A time and motion study in 4 specialties. *Annals of Internal Medicine, 165*(11), 753–760. https://doi.org/10.7326/M16-0961.
    - The time-and-motion study demonstrated the disproportionate time clinicians spend on administrative tasks relative to patient care.

7. Rotenstein, L. S., Torre, M., Ramos, M. A., Rosales, R. C., Guille, C., Sen, S., and Mata, D. A. (2018). Prevalence of burnout among physicians: A systematic review. *JAMA, 320*(11), 1131–1150. https://doi.org/10.1001/jama.2018.12777.
    - A review article focusing on physician burnout due to current clinical workflow inefficiencies and administrative burdens.

8. Wrenn, J. O., Stein, D. M., Bakken, S., and Stetson, P. D. (2010). Quantifying clinical narrative redundancy in an electronic health record. *Journal of the American Medical Informatics Association, 17*(1), 49–53. https://doi.org/10.1197/jamia.M3390.
    - Highlights the risks associated with "copy-and-paste" functionality in electronic health records, including the potential for errors and reduced data quality.

LLMs and NLP in healthcare

9. Yang, X., Chen, A., PourNejatian, N., Shin, H. C., Smith, K. E., Parisien, C., Compas, C., Martin, C., Flores, M. G., Zhang, Y., Magoc, T., Harle, C. A., Lipori, G., Mitchell, D. A., Hogan, W. R., Shenkman, E. A., Bian, J., and Wu, Y. (2022). arXiv preprint arXiv:2203.03540. Available at: https://arxiv.org/abs/2203.03540.
    - This study introduces GatorTron, a large clinical language model developed to process unstructured electronic health records

(EHRs), aiming to enhance healthcare delivery by extracting valuable patient information.

10. Matos, J., Gallifant, J., Pei, J., and Wong, A. I. (2024). EHRmonize: A framework for medical concept abstraction from electronic health records using large language models. arXiv preprint arXiv:2407.00242. Available at: from https://arxiv.org/abs/2407.00242.

   • This research presents EHRmonize, a framework that leverages LLMs to abstract medical concepts from EHR data, thereby improving data harmonization and facilitating healthcare research.

11. Haltaufderheide, J. and Ranisch, R. (2024). The ethics of ChatGPT in medicine and healthcare: A systematic review on large language models (LLMs). *arXiv preprint arXiv:2403.14473.* Available at: https://arxiv.org/abs/2403.14473.

   • This systematic review examines the ethical considerations associated with deploying LLMs such as ChatGPT in medical and healthcare settings, discussing potential benefits and ethical challenges.

Impact on provider workflows and patient experiences

12. Obermeyer, Z., Powers, B., Vogeli, C., and Mullainathan, S. (2019). Dissecting racial bias in an algorithm used to manage the health of populations. *Science, 366*(6464), 447–453. https://doi.org/10.1126/science.aax2342.

   • Analyzes how AI, including LLMs, can introduce or mitigate biases in clinical workflows and affect patient outcomes.

13. Rajpurkar, P., Chen, E., Banerjee, O., and Topol, E. J. (2022). AI in health and medicine. *Nature Medicine, 28*(1), 31–38. https://doi.org/10.1038/s41591-021-01614-0.

   • Provides a state-of-the-art review of AI, particularly LLMs, in improving patient–provider interactions and democratizing healthcare.

Future directions and ethical considerations

14. Bhayana, R., Krishna, S., and Bleakney, R. (2023). Performance of ChatGPT on a radiology board-style examination: Insights into current strengths and limitations. *Radiology, 307*(1), e230582. https://doi.org/10.1148/radiol.230582.

- Evaluates ChatGPT's performance on radiology exam questions, shedding light on its potential and limitations in clinical education and decision-making.
15. Leslie, D. (2019). Understanding artificial intelligence ethics and safety: A guide for the responsible design and implementation of AI systems in the public sector. *The Alan Turing Institute.* Available at: https://www.turing.ac.uk/news/publications/understanding-artificial-intelligence-ethics-and-safety.
   - Explores the ethical frameworks and considerations for deploying AI systems in the public sector.
16. Floridi, L. and Cowls, J. (2019). A unified framework of five principles for AI in society. *Harvard Data Science Review, 1*(1), 1–13. https://doi.org/10.1162/99608f92.8cd550d1.
   - Discusses ethical principles for AI and the notion of explicability.

https://doi.org/10.1142/9789819813506_0004

Chapter 4

Healthcare Goes Digital: Toward the Collaborative Digital Transformation Approach

Leonardo Caporarello and Iuliia Trabskaia

Bocconi University and SDA Bocconi School of Management, Milan, Italy

1. Introduction

Healthcare faces many challenges with the significant aging of the population and the need for appropriate treatment, increased competition including the emergence of new players on the market, supply chain issues, demand for customization, personalization, and new customer experiences (Preko *et al.*, 2020; Svensson *et al.*, 2021; Beaulieu and Bentahar, 2021).

Today, digital transformation has emerged as an effective opportunity to overcome the abovementioned challenges in healthcare. Digitalization has affected many aspects of healthcare, including administration, service delivery, patient experience, and prognostic capabilities (Vaagan *et al.*, 2021; Senbekov *et al.*, 2020). Indeed, digital tools such as cloud-based electronic health records, nanotechnology-enabled devices, telemedicine platforms, AI (e.g., AI-based prediction and diagnostics), e-Health, and robots (e.g., virtual assistants) are emerging in healthcare.

Although promising, digital transformation often remains incomplete, fragmented, with many barriers and risks (Kho *et al.*, 2020). In this context, healthcare is pushed to further adopt digital innovation.

Certainly, digital transformation brings numerous advantages and opportunities to healthcare and should continue to be implemented (Ghosh *et al.*, 2023). However, along with the benefits, digital transformation poses challenges. Diverse barriers arise at the organizational level from both employees' and patients' point of view. From the employees' perspectives, barriers include employee skills gap, resistance to innovation, lack of understanding regarding the purpose of digitalization, and fear of replacement. From the patients' perspectives, there is resistance to innovation and lack of skills to effectively use digital tools. Furthermore, difficulties arise both at the organizational level and at the industry level. The healthcare ecosystem is highly complex, with its various stakeholders inextricably linked, making digital transformation challenging. Harmonization and coordinated efforts are essential to navigate this complexity successfully. Furthermore, there are other challenges of digital transformation related to the ethical aspects of patient data, data security, and data privacy (Jahankhani and Kendzierskyj, 2019).

However, researchers and practitioners agree that among all challenges, the most significant barriers to digitalization of healthcare lie in the resource's limitations (Blix and Levay, 2018; Gjellebæk *et al.*, 2020; Kruse *et al.*, 2018), including financial, human, and expertise.

To overcome this barrier, much can be realized through collaborative digital transformation. Collaboration allows to get access to the partner's resources, experience, and knowledge. So far, collaboration has become an influential strategy for the adoption of organizational innovations including digital transformation.

Despite the importance of collaboration as a driver of company development and digital transformation, the significance of collaborative digital transformation is still underreported in the literature. Especially little attention has been paid to the impact of collaborations on digital transformation in the healthcare sector. Just a few authors examine collaborations in the context of digital transformation in healthcare (e.g., Balta *et al.*, 2021; Kryzhanivska *et al.*, 2025).

This chapter aims to close this gap in the literature and analyze how collaborations are driving digital transformation and how collaborative digital transformation can serve as an effective model for addressing challenges while creating value for all stakeholders, including patients and society at large, within healthcare settings. The research questions are as follows: (1) How is collaborative digital transformation adopted in healthcare? (2) How do different stakeholders benefit from collaborative digital transformation? This chapter is based on case studies of companies. The case studies provide a nuanced examination of collaborative digital transformation in healthcare.

This chapter is structured as follows: It begins with a literature review on digital transformation in healthcare, providing a foundation for understanding the key trends and challenges in the sector. This is followed by a section on collaborations, exploring their role in driving innovation and overcoming barriers to digital transformation. Next, this chapter presents a description of the research methodology. The results of the research are then presented. This chapter concludes with a discussion, summarizing the key findings and suggesting potential directions for future research.

2. Digital Transformation in Healthcare

Digital transformation has fundamentally changed the healthcare industry. "The digital revolution in healthcare creates new business opportunities and yields new business models to address issues in medical practice, value creation and other problems related to, among others, the ageing society" (Kraus *et al.*, 2020, p. 1). For example, the AI-in-healthcare market has achieved significant growth and is expected to grow further at a global level to an estimated $45.2 billion by 2026 (Samavedam, 2024).

Indeed, the prospects for the development of the healthcare industry, the creation of a new value proposition, new services, and improvements in quality are vast. Digital transformation increases the accessibility of healthcare for different population groups, including those with limited mobility and those living at a distance, and healthcare inequalities (Raimo *et al.*, 2023). Furthermore, digital transformation enhances both the speed and quality of services for patients (Agarwal *et al.*, 2010). It creates significant opportunities to improve healthcare service delivery, offering various approaches to optimize patient care, including consumerization strategies, e.g., ePrescription, which does not require the patient to spend time visiting a doctor for a prescription but is fast enough to get a prescription online. There are other value-added services, such as home testing, chatbots, and digital assistants (Gopal *et al.*, 2019).

Furthermore, big data and data analytics provide great predictive capabilities (e.g., Intelligent Diagnostics). Incorporation of data from different sources allows for keeping a long-term history of a patient's health status and improving the decision-making process of medical staff based on data analysis. For example, in Estonia, the Genome Centre aimed to collect data from Estonian residents and create a genomic repository. The repository contains data on oncological diseases of women, focusing on whether their ancestors had such diseases. On the basis of data from the repository, a forecast of the threat of oncology is created and preventive measures are proposed (the frequency of the need for tests, tests, etc.).

Above all, AI-driven healthcare is emerging as a distinct phenomenon, bringing a number of breakthroughs including tracking, monitoring, and predictive capabilities (Zahlan *et al*., 2023). Among others, AI-driven technologies provide significant financial benefits; in this vein, according to a McKinsey report, "AI, traditional machine learning, and deep learning are projected to result in net savings of up to $360 billion in healthcare spending" (Eastburn *et al*., 2024, p. 1).

Digital transformation also brings benefits to healthcare staff, as much of the routine work of administrative staff can now be automated. Additionally, digitalization opens a wide range of opportunities for digital training and development of staff.

However, despite all the opportunities offered by digital transformation, there are several barriers to its implementation and adoption processes. These include the resistance to innovation (Haider and Kreps, 2004; Cannavale *et al*., 2023), the digital skills gap of employees, the fear of replacement with technology, the speed of introduction of technologies, the transformation of the consumer experience, the need to change the business model, and others.

There are also several complexities unique to healthcare, as noted by Hermes *et al*. (2019). Foremost is the multilevel and multiagents' structure of the healthcare ecosystem, which includes patients, public and private hospitals, insurance companies, suppliers, policymakers, and more. Given the tightly interconnected nature of these relationships, digitalization efforts must be harmonized among all actors within the ecosystem. Further, researchers have reported the problem of personal health information security (Fichman *et al*., 2011), since the health data of a patient is very sensitive, and its disclosure is extremely sensitive. Consequently, this must be considered during digitalization.

In addition to the above-mentioned difficulties, COVID has put pressure on the healthcare system, which has made the digital transformation urgent (Dal Mas *et al.*, 2023). The pandemic required dramatic organizational changes affecting different parts of the industry, including the introduction of telehealth, supply-chain interactions, and medical teleconsultation platforms. However, due to the urgency, the digital transformation was often fragmented, lacking a systematic approach.

All these challenges pushed healthcare managers to rethink strategy, including searching for new resources and solutions. One of the promising strategic directions for the further development of digital transformation in healthcare lies in the adoption of a collaborative strategy which fosters innovation and resource sharing across stakeholders.

3. Collaborative Digital Transformation

As described above, a range of factors and trends in today's rapidly changing environment are pushing healthcare industry organizations to further digital transformation. However, the healthcare industry faces a number of significant barriers along the way of digitalization. The most important limitation is the shortage of resources and capabilities within organizations. Among the resources and capabilities that are limited in healthcare, we can mention, among others, financial resources (for example, expertise in obtaining grants and funding), technological skills, and expertise in driving innovation.

Previous literature suggests that collaboration plays a crucial role in overcoming resource limitations (Teece, 1986; Bettiol *et al.*, 2023). This is because collaboration involves the sharing of resources, expertise, knowledge, experience, and reputation. As a result, collaboration offers significant benefits to all parties involved, as they pool their resources and complement each other's strengths to achieve shared objectives (Carbonara and Pellegrino, 2020).

The Network Theory (e.g., Bennett *et al.*, 2008) provides a theoretical foundation for this dynamic, emphasizing that networking leads to sharing activities, information, and insights. This synergy yields high-value outcomes for all parties involved, demonstrating the impact of collaborative efforts on innovation.

Moreover, collaboration allows sharing risks and reducing the degree of uncertainty. Losses can also be reduced as a consequence of the collaboration since solutions to mitigate losses can be found through a collaborative approach. Furthermore, collaboration will allow us to reconfigure the business model and develop a more efficient development strategy (Belitski and Mariani, 2023).

In addition to the above arguments explaining the benefits of collaboration, it is essential to recognize that collaboration is a powerful driver of innovation. Collaboration facilitates the sharing of knowledge, expertise, and experience, creating a more robust intellectual pool where each participant reinforces the others. Furthermore, collaborations often involve interdisciplinarity, when both internal and external partners can be part of collaborative efforts. This cross-disciplinary exchange fosters the development of innovative projects that combine expertise from various fields.

Collaboration brings a whole stream of benefits to both collaborators and other groups of stakeholders. For example, collaboration brings social benefits to the state, different groups of the population, businesses (e.g., they provide models of collaboration that other companies can adopt), patients, and employees of the healthcare sector.

In the context of digital transformation, the benefits and impact of collaboration align with the arguments mentioned above. The issue of resource limitation is particularly pressing in digital transformation. It is evident that such transformation requires significant financial investment, and technical resources, as well as a deep understanding of how best to adopt digital innovations. Moreover, digital transformation demands a new set of capabilities and often even new business models (Molla and Bhalla, 2006). Under these conditions, collaborative digital transformation can offer an effective model. This is especially true in the healthcare sector, where ensuring high-quality outcomes is crucial, and where combining the expertise of healthcare professionals with digital specialists is essential.

However, the study of collaborative digital transformation and its effects remains an underexplored area, particularly within healthcare. While collaborations in healthcare have received some attention from researchers, they have typically been considered outside the scope of digital transformation. Previous studies have focused more on interprofessional and interorganizational collaboration (e.g., Morley and Cashell, 2017; Karam *et al.*, 2018; van der Schors *et al.*, 2021), without fully addressing the transformative potential of digital innovation within these partnerships. In this vein, in a recent extensive literature review (Dal Mas *et al.*, 2023), the authors found that collaborations were not identified as a significant focus within the existing body of research on digital transformation in healthcare.

4. Research Design

Following the above, this chapter aims to research how collaborative digital transformation models are implemented in healthcare settings, and by examining the benefits, these models bring to both collaborators and other stakeholders. This research is based on a case study approach. The case methodology was chosen since it provides an opportunity to understand the essence of the phenomenon in depth and in detail, to trace the process and the point of view of all stakeholders qualitatively (Alam, 2021). Case studies are valuable tools for exploring complex issues through detailed, contextual analysis. By examining real-life situations in depth, case studies provide a rich understanding of how specific concepts or strategies are applied in practice.

In the context of this research, the case studies aim to identify how collaboration processes are driving digital transformation in healthcare. The most important tasks are to identify what problem the collaboration solved and what benefits the collaboration brought to the collaborators and other stakeholders, including the healthcare industry as a whole. Also, it is important in this research to understand why "collaboration" is useful for healthcare management today and in the future, collaborations that would make a practical contribution for businesses and educators.

First, a key source of information on collaborations in healthcare and digital transformation was selected. The European Digital Innovation Hubs Network grant program was chosen as such a source based on several criteria:

- The thematic focus on digital innovation, which fully coincides with the topic of this chapter and its research questions: (1) How is collaborative digital transformation adopted in healthcare? (2) How do different stakeholders benefit from collaborative digital transformation?
- The European Digital Innovation Hubs Network grant program is highly prestigious, with rigorous requirements and criteria for selecting projects and participants. As a result, the projects approved under this

grant are characterized by their exceptional quality and the thorough development of concepts, strategies, and other key components.

- From the timeline perspective, it is a modern grant, as many projects have been implemented or have completed the first stage of project implementation under the grant in autumn 2024.
- There are already project results within the framework of this grant, and they can be evaluated and analyzed.
- An important indicator of success in this grant is the social impact on different groups of stakeholders.
- Many of the grant projects are based on collaborations.

As part of this grant program, we selected case studies based on several key criteria:

- connection with the healthcare sector,
- focus on digital transformation,
- collaborative projects.

A total of 109 projects were presented within the grant program, 20 of which were dedicated to healthcare, and 2 projects fully met the criteria of our study (see Table 1).

Table 1.   Cases for analysis.

Project title	Link	Collaborators
From Concept to Innovation: How EDIH.SH guided AIcendence to Success in Healthcare	https://european-digital-innovation-hubs.ec.europa.eu/knowledge-hub/success-stories/concept-innovation-how-edihsh-guided-aicendence-success-healthcare	• EDIH.SH consulting company • Start-up AIcendence (AI technology in the healthcare sector)
Collaboration Promises to Revolutionize Healthcare Education	https://european-digital-innovation-hubs.ec.europa.eu/knowledge-hub/success-stories/collaboration-promises-revolutionise-healthcare-education	• ThingLink platform • the University of Eastern Finland • Kuopio Health

Cases analysis framework is partially based on the structure outlined in The European Digital Innovation Hubs (European Commission, 2024):

- *Organizations-collaborators*: An overview of the organizations involved in the collaboration, including their roles and contributions.
- *Identification of the problem*: A clear outline of the key challenges or issues that prompted the collaboration.
- *Essence of the collaboration*: An examination of the nature and structure of the collaboration, including the goals, processes, and interactions between partners.
- *Benefits to the parties involved*: A detailed look at how each participant in the collaboration benefited from their involvement.
- *Benefits to society and other stakeholders*: An assessment of the broader impact of the collaboration on society and other relevant stakeholders.

This framework will guide our analysis and help uncover the dynamics, outcomes, and broader implications of collaborative efforts in the healthcare sector, particularly in the context of digital transformation.

5. Results

5.1. *Case 1. From concept to innovation: How EDIH.SH guided AIcendence to success in healthcare*

Organizations-collaborators: The first case is *From Concept to Innovation: How EDIH.SH guided AIcendence to Success in Healthcare*. The collaboration involved the following: (1) EDIH.SH, a company with a reputation and a long history of excellence in e-commerce and healthcare system requirements, and (2) AIcendence, an AI-driven startup offering AI solutions for healthcare.

Identification of the problem: This case study is particularly interesting because the focus shifts away from traditional healthcare providers and centers on a tech startup. The startup, which offers an AI-driven solution called Cyto-ML, developed a product designed to revolutionize healthcare diagnostics. *Cyto-ML* is not only significantly more accurate but also 30 times faster than conventional methods, promising patients quicker and more reliable diagnoses. However, the startup faced the challenge of expressing the value of its innovative technology within the healthcare field.

Essence of the collaboration: The collaboration consisted of AIcendence startup contributing its startup idea and expertise. EDIH.SH company contributes its expertise in healthcare-related legislation in the EU, including Medical Device Regulation (MDR). EDIH.SH also assisted with grant applications, bureaucratic procedures, legislative requirements, etc.

Benefits to the parties involved: AIcendence received expert support in legislative issues of the healthcare sector, support in obtaining a grant, and general support in legislative requirements for the implementation of their startup idea, for bringing the company to the market, and for scaling their business and attracting further investments. So far, the benefits of AIcendence startup are mostly financial, market-related, and strategical.

EDIH.SH gained substantial reputational benefits from this collaboration, notably through the expansion of its portfolio of successful consulting projects. Particularly valuable was their involvement in implementing AI solutions – technologies that are in high demand today. This not only enhanced their standing as a key player in the tech-consulting space but also positioned them as a critical enabler of innovation within the healthcare sector.

Benefits to society and other stakeholders: Obviously, the society gets a whole range of benefits, such as the application technology, which allows making diagnostics more accurate and with less resources. Also, an important benefit is the collaboration model, where startups are supported by consulting companies. This collaborative digital transformation model also plays a vital role in strengthening the broader innovation system by offering a valuable framework for supporting and commercializing innovations. By bringing together diverse stakeholders and leveraging their complementary expertise, the collaboration helps bridge the gap between research and market application, facilitating the successful translation of new technologies into practical solutions.

Additionally, the collaboration contributes to the business community by fostering the development of an innovative business model. This new model not only enhances the efficiency of bringing AI-driven solutions to market (for different groups of stakeholders) but also opens new opportunities for entrepreneurs (to apply this model).

5.2. Case 2. Collaboration promises to revolutionize healthcare education

Organizations-collaborators: HealthHub Finland EDIH's 'Test before invest' services, ThingLink platform, is an AI-based content creator, the University of Eastern Finland, and Kuopio Health participated in the collaboration.

Identification of the problem: First is for universities to create interesting content considering the needs of modern consumers (e.g., consumers' demands to make courses more interactive, visual, arousing curiosity, and less academic). Second, for universities, there is the problem of digital literacy of professors. In general, there is a demand for a high-quality modern contest in the health sector.

Essence of the collaboration: The collaboration allowed the development of the AI tool ThingLink for the design of user-friendly courses in healthcare. This tool helped transform a typical healthcare course that was full of materials, papers, and text into a more digestible experience based on the principles of modern educational model, such as interactivity, creativity, arousal of curiosity, and development of creative thinking.

Benefits to the parties involved: For the ThingLink platform, the collaboration allows them to show the high quality of their product, to promote their position in the market, and to show the full capabilities of their AI-based content creator. For universities, the major benefit is represented by the possibility of delivering a high-quality and high-engaging course with content that responds to the behavioral patterns of modern students. Moreover, universities can improve the quality of education and increase student satisfaction with the overall learning experience.

Benefits to society and other stakeholders: First, there is a contribution to the society, including consumers, as it is an educational program accessible (e.g., for people from different geographical areas, with different languages). Second, a significant impact is made on the health sector itself. In this vein, such easily created and accessible courses contribute to the growth of the quality of training, lead to a reduction in resource costs (financial, human, and time), and improve learning outcomes. Third, the product of collaborative efforts brings benefits for educators because the

AI tool does not require special knowledge of tools (such as program-ming) to create a course, i.e., a teacher who has expertise in healthcare does not have to have expertise in technology. So far, educators with even limited digital literacy have been able to easily upload their materials, such as texts, into the AI tool.

6. Conclusion and Discussion

Healthcare, in light of modern challenges, is in urgent need of further digi-tal transformation. While digital transformation offers numerous benefits to the sector as a whole and to individual organizations, it also presents a range of barriers and risks. Among the most significant obstacles are limited resources – both financial and human – as well as the need for specialized skills and capabilities.

As highlighted in previous research (Ang, 2008; Dockx, 2023), col-laboration represents an effective tool for driving innovation, including digital transformation. A key mechanism fostering innovation is the exchange of resources, information, knowledge, and experience that takes place during collaborative efforts (Levine and Prietula, 2014). According to networking theory (e.g., Borgatti and Halgin, 2011), collaborative net-works facilitate the efficient exchange of ideas, knowledge, and insights. The interdisciplinary nature of such collaborations further enhances their potential by bringing together diverse perspectives and expertise from different sectors.

Thus, based on the points outlined above, collaborative digital trans-formation emerges as a promising approach that allows participants to leverage each other's strengths, thereby accelerating the digital transfor-mation process and overcoming resource constraints.

In this study, we have analyzed cases of collaborative digital transfor-mation between healthcare organizations and organizations from other sectors. As a basis, we took projects selected within the framework of a reputable European grant focused on the most successful digital innova-tion projects. Within the framework of the grant, we identified two cases in which successful digital transformation was achieved through collab-orative efforts.

In one case, the collaborative digital transformation made possible the successful development of a consulting company and a startup in the healthcare sector, as a result of which the AI innovation was brought to the market and successfully implemented. This project has brought a number of benefits to both collaborators and other stakeholders.

The second case study involves the collaborative digital transformation of a technology platform and universities, as an output of the collaboration, a tool for AI to create interactive and useful courses in the health sector was developed. This project has also added benefits to both the collaborators and other stakeholders.

The theoretical contribution of this study lies in advancing our understanding of collaborative transformation by introducing the concept of collaborative digital transformation in healthcare. To the best of our knowledge, this is the first time that collaborative digital transformation has been explored as a model for effective change, especially in the healthcare sector. Additionally, the contribution of this study lies in examining the role of collaborative digital transformation as a key driver of benefits, not only for the collaborators themselves but also for other stakeholders.

The practical implication of this research is to highlight how collaborative digital transformation models can be applied across healthcare settings. The collaborative models and strategies analyzed in this study offer insights that can help healthcare organizations improve their innovation capacity and, at the same time, optimize their resources. Moreover, the research shows how collaboration addresses barriers (resource limitations) and drives innovation. As such, the findings can serve as a useful instrument for healthcare organizations that provide guidance on how to apply collaborative approaches to address the challenges of digital transformation.

This study has several limitations. One key limitation is that the cases analyzed focus only on certain stakeholders within the healthcare ecosystem, specifically startups, universities, and consulting companies. Future research could broaden the scope by including a wider range of stakeholders, such as government bodies, public and private hospitals, medical equipment producers, and other relevant actors involved in healthcare collaboration. Another limitation of this study is its static approach to examining the impact of collaborations on digital transformation and the development of collaborative digital transformation. The research examines the effects of collaborations at a single point in time rather than exploring the process from a dynamic perspective. It would be interesting to trace how collaborative digital transformation evolves over time to better understand how they stimulate digital transformation and the dynamics of this impact.

References

Alam, M. K. (2021). A systematic qualitative case study: Questions, data collection, NVivo analysis and saturation. *Qualitative Research in Organizations and Management: An International Journal, 16*(1), 1–31.

Agarwal, R., Gao, G., DesRoches, C., and Jha, A. K. (2010). Research commentary – The digital transformation of healthcare: Current status and the road ahead. *Information Systems Research, 21*(4), 796–809.

Ang, S. H. (2008). Competitive intensity and collaboration: Impact on firm growth across technological environments. *Strategic Management Journal, 29*(10), 1057–1075. https://doi.org/10.1002/smj.695.

Beaulieu, M. and Bentahar, O. (2021). Digitalization of the healthcare supply chain: A roadmap to generate benefits and effectively support healthcare delivery. *Technological Forecasting and Social Change, 167*, 120717.

Balta, M., Valsecchi, R., Papadopoulos, T., and Bourne, D. J. (2021). Digitalization and co-creation of healthcare value: A case study in Occupational Health. *Technological Forecasting and Social Change, 168*, 120785.

Belitski, M. and Mariani, M. (2023). The effect of knowledge collaboration on business model reconfiguration. *European Management Journal, 41*(2), 223–235.

Bennett, J. (2018). Whose place is this anyway? An actor-network theory exploration of a conservation conflict. *Space and Culture, 21*(2), 159–169.

Bettiol, M., Capestro, M., DiMaria, E., and Grandinetti, R. (2023). Leveraging on intra- and inter-organizational collaboration in industry 4.0 adoption for knowledge creation and innovation. *European Journal of Innovation Management, 26*(7), 328–352. https://doi.org/10.1108/ejim-10-2022-0593.

Blix, M. and Levay, C. (2018). Digitalization and health care. *Eso expertgrupp, 44*, 13–35.

Borgatti, S. P. and Halgin, D. S. (2011). On network theory. *Organization Science, 22*(5), 1168–1181.

Carbonara, N. and Pellegrino, R. (2020). The role of public private partnerships in fostering innovation. *Construction Management and Economics, 38*(2), 140–156.

Dal Mas, F., Massaro, M., Rippa, P., and Secundo, G. (2023). The challenges of digital transformation in healthcare: An interdisciplinary literature review, framework, and future research agenda. *Technovation, 123*, 102716.

Dockx, E., Verhoest, K., Langbroek, T., and Wynen, J. (2023). Bringing together unlikely innovators: do connective and learning capacities impact collaboration for innovation and diversity of actors? *Public Management Review, 25*(6), 1104–1127.

Eastburn, J., Fowkes, J., Kellner, K., and Swanson, B. (2024). Digital Transformation: Health Systems' Investment Priorities. McKinsey

European Commission. (2024). The European Digital Innovation Hubs. https:// european-digital-innovation-hubs.ec.europa.eu/get-know-us.

Fichman, G., Kohli, R., and Krishnan, R. (2011). The role of information systems in healthcare: Current research and future trends. *Information Systems Research, 22,* 419–327. http://dx.doi.org/10.1287/isre.1110.0382.

Gjellebæk, C., Svensson, A., Bjørkquist, C., Fladeby, N., and Grundén, K. (2020). Management challenges for future digitalization of healthcare services. *Futures, 124,* 102636.

Ghosh, K., Dohan, M. S., Veldandi, H., and Garfield, M. (2023). Digital transformation in healthcare: Insights on value creation. *Journal of Computer Information Systems, 63*(2), 449–459.

Gopal, G., Suter-Crazzolara, C., Toldo, L., and Eberhardt, W. (2019). Digital transformation in healthcare–architectures of present and future information technologies. *Clinical Chemistry and Laboratory Medicine* (CCLM), *57*(3), 328–335.

Haider, M. and Kreps, G. L. (2004). Forty years of diffusion of innovations: Utility and value in public health. *Journal of Health Communication, 9*(S1), 3–11.

Jahankhani, H. and Kendzierskyj, S. (2019). Digital transformation of healthcare. *Blockchain and Clinical Trial: Securing Patient Data,* pp. 31–52. Springer, Cham, Switzerland.

Karam, M., Brault, I., Van Durme, T., and Macq, J. (2018). Comparing interprofessional and interorganizational collaboration in healthcare: A systematic review of the qualitative research. *International Journal of Nursing Studies, 79,* 70–83.

Kho, J., Gillespie, N., and Martin-Khan, M. (2020). A systematic scoping review of change management practices used for telemedicine service implementations. *BMC Health Services Research, 2*0, 1–16.

Kraus, S., Schiavone, F., Pluzhnikova, A., and Invernizzi, A. C. (2021). Digital transformation in healthcare: Analyzing the current state-of-research. *Journal of Business Research, 123,* 557–567.

Kryzhanivska, K., Albats, E., Blomqvist, K., and Mention, A. L. (2024). Transforming inter-organisational collaboration dynamics in regional networks through digitalisation. *Regional Studies, 59*(1), 1–17.

Kruse, C. S., Karem, P., Shifflett, K., Vegi, L., Ravi, K., and Brooks, M. (2018). Evaluating barriers to adopting telemedicine worldwide: A systematic review. *Journal of Telemedicine and Telecare, 24*(1), 4–12.

Levine, S. S. and Prietula, M. J. (2014). Open collaboration for innovation: Principles and performance. *Organization Science, 25*(5), 1414–1433.

Molla, A. and Bhalla, A. (2006). Business transformation through ERP: A case study of an Asian company. *Journal of Information Technology Case and Application Research, 8*(1), 34–54.

Morley, L. and Cashell, A. (2017). Collaboration in health care. *Journal of Medical Imaging and Radiation Sciences*, *48*(2), 207–216.

Preko, M., Osei-Boateng, R., and Durosinmi, A. E. (2020). Digitalising health-care in developing economies: Challenges and mitigating strategies. In *Handbook of Research on Managing Information Systems in Developing Economies*, pp. 332–353, IGI Global, USA, Pennsylvania.

Raimo, N., De Turi, I., Albergo, F., and Vitolla, F. (2023). The drivers of the digi-tal transformation in the healthcare industry: An empirical analysis in Italian hospitals. *Technovation, 121*, 102558.

Samavedam, R. (2024). Inclusive Innovation: Key to the Future of Healthcare.

Senbekov, M., Saliev, T., Bukeyeva, Z., Almabayeva, A., Zhanaliyeva, M., Aitenova, N., Toishibekov, Y., and Fakhradiyev, I. (2020). The recent prog-ress and applications of digital technologies in healthcare: A review. *International Journal of Telemedicine and Applications*, *2020*(1), 8830200.

Svensson, A., Bergkvist, L., Bäccman, C., and Durst, S. (2021). Challenges in implementing digital assistive technology in municipal healthcare. In *Management and Information Technology after Digital Transformation*. Routledge, pp. 81–90. Milton Park, Abingdon-on-Thames, Oxfordshire, England, UK.

Teece, D. J. (1986). Profiting from technological innovation: Implications for integration, collaboration, licensing and public policy. *Research Policy*, *15*(6), 285–305.

Vaagan, R. W., Torkkola, S., Sendra, A., Farré, J., and Lovari, A. (2021). A critical analysis of the digitization of healthcare communication in the EU: A com-parison of Italy, Finland, Norway, and Spain. *International Journal of Communication*, *15*, 23.

van der Schors, W., Roos, A. F., Kemp, R., and Varkevisser, M. (2021). Inter-organizational collaboration between healthcare providers. *Health Services Management Research, 34*(1), 36–46.

Zahlan, A., Ranjan, R. P., and Hayes, D. (2023). Artificial intelligence innovation in healthcare: Literature review, exploratory analysis, and future research. *Technology in Society, 74*, 102321.

https://doi.org/10.1142/9789819813506_0005

Chapter 5

Digital Transformation of Healthcare Facility Management Services

Paul Schmitter

ZHAW School of Life Sciences and
Facility Management, Switzerland

1. Introduction

The ongoing digital disruption is reshaping the healthcare system, including medical and care services, as well as the non-medical support services of which facility management (FM) is part of. Digitalization presents significant opportunities for FM services to achieve organizational, sustainability, and financial objectives (Redlein and Höhenberger, 2020). The advantages of digital FM are well documented in the literature. These include improved cost performance (Huynh and Nguyen-Ky, 2020), enhanced building sustainability (Lavikka *et al.*, 2017), better building performance (Godager *et al.*, 2021), increased productivity, and service efficiency (Lok *et al.*, 2023), automation of building systems, real-time building condition information, and predictive maintenance (Hakimi *et al.*, 2024). Digital technologies can also enhance occupant experience, safety and security, and workplace productivity and foster collaboration and skills development.

Despite the potential, the FM industry has lagged behind others in terms of digital adoption rate, reflected in the low digital maturity levels as reported by Pedral Sampaio *et al.* (2023). This situation also applies to FM in healthcare, where significant efforts are required to bridge the current digital gap. Implementing such digital technologies poses significant challenges for FM. Especially within healthcare organizations, such as hospitals, a highly complex environment with various stakeholders requires careful coordination. Rather than focusing on digital solutions alone, structural changes and an effective approach to technology adoption are essential. This requires a comprehensive understanding of digitalization and digital transformation that extends beyond the typical scope of digital FM.

2. Facility Management in Healthcare

The built environment of healthcare organizations is among some of the most complex. In most cases, healthcare facilities must be operated continuously 24/7 with minimal or no downtime. Furthermore, the core medical and care services in a healthcare organization, such as a hospital, elderly care home, or clinic, require additional support services in order to provide patients and residents optimal health care. In this regard, FM provides a wide range of non-medical support services, critical for the built environment and core healthcare activities. In healthcare institutions, especially complex ones, such as hospitals, FM-related services account for around a third of costs (Lennerts *et al.*, 2003). In addition, FM plays a critical role in the design, planning, and construction phases of infrastructure and therefore has a high leverage effect on the subsequent operational expenditure (OPEX). The implementation of well-designed healthcare buildings that meet the specified operational requirements can directly reduce costs throughout a healthcare-buildings' life cycle (Lavy and Terzioğlu, 2023; Lerzynski, 2021; Sampaio *et al.*, 2023; Wang *et al.*, 2013). A further crucial aspect where FM services have a high significance is in patient satisfaction. The perception of the quality of the physical and social environment influences that of the medical and care services (Gerber *et al.*, 2020). As a service management discipline, the service-oriented perspective of FM (Coenen and Von Felten, 2014) is a clear advantage. In this regard, FM is of great importance for healthcare organizations.

2.1. *Definition*

The International Organization for Standardization (ISO) (2017) defines FM as an "organizational function which integrates people, place and process [...] within the built environment [...] with the purpose of improving the quality [...] of life of people and the productivity of the core business." FM thus ensures that the necessary services, spaces, and infrastructure meet the requirements that enable the primary activities. Nutt (1999) asserts that FM functions integrate the physical, human, and financial areas of a business. Facility managers must translate the needs of the core business into spaces, infrastructures, and services. As a multidisciplinary business function and managerial role, FM operates on strategic, tactical, and operational level, ensuring all requirements between clients and suppliers are met (Paliderova and Michalikova, 2018). Lavy and Shohet (2007) defined the so-called healthcare FM as a strategic and operational management discipline of non-medical activities for healthcare facilities. Primary areas include maintenance management, energy and operations, performance and risk management, and business management and development. However, the scope of FM in healthcare extends beyond the technical aspects of the built environment, to include soft services, such as catering, hygiene, cleaning, textile supply, or hotel services (Hofer and Gerber, 2015).

2.2. *Scope and services*

Due to its interdisciplinary nature, greater complexity, and broader scope of specialized services, FM in the healthcare sector cannot be compared to its implementations in other industries. Under the umbrella of non-medical support services, Gerber and Kuchen (2019) provide a clear frame of reference, as presented in Figure 1, that positions, outlines, and lists the relevant services. The associated Service Catalogue for Non-medical Services in Hospitals is also a valuable instrument for the definition and specification of service provision in healthcare organizations. Although the allocation model and service catalogs were developed specifically for hospitals, the application can be adapted in all relevant healthcare organizations where non-medical services are provided.

The model by Gerber and Kuchen (2019) distinguishes core services, support services, and management services. Core services are medical

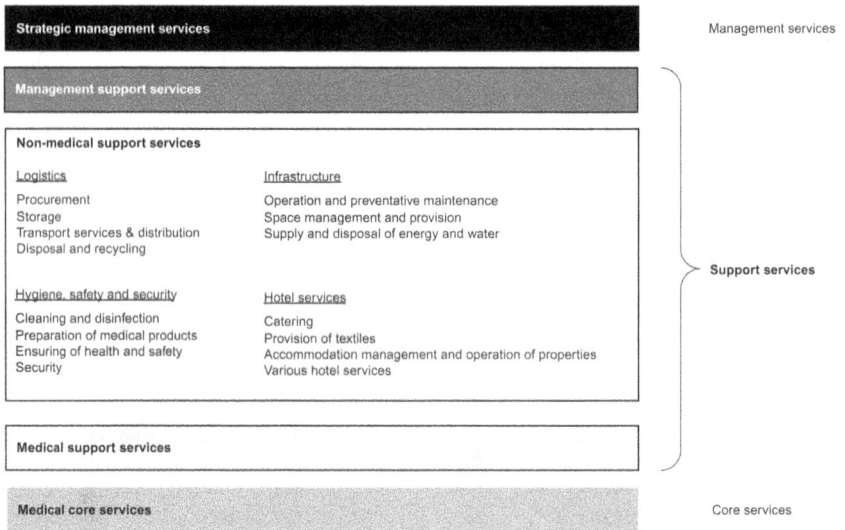

Figure 1.   Allocation model of medical and non-medical services in hospitals.

Source: Adapted from *Service Catalogue for Non-medical Services in Hospitals (LekaS): Version 2.0: Translation of the German Original*, by Gerber and Kuchen (2019, p. 10).

services, consisting of diagnostics, therapy, and nursing care. Support services are further delineated into three categories:

i. medical support services, which include areas such as pharmacy, laboratory, and related clinical functions,
ii. non-medical support services, encompassing logistics, infrastructure, hygiene, security, and hospitality services,
iii. management support services, covering key operational domains, such as finance, controlling, and human resource management.

Finally, overarching both core and support services are the strategic management services, which integrate critical elements, such as sustainability, quality management, and other long-term organizational imperatives. The scope of non-medical support services operates primarily at the tactical and operational levels within the model. However, their impact extends beyond operational and tactical domains, influencing both management and strategic services. This is why Hofer and Gerber (2015) proposed to introduce Chief Facility Managing Officers (CFMOs) who are present at the board level. The necessity for the strategic relevance of

FM can be seen in areas such as sustainability, quality management, risk management, sourcing, asset, and portfolio strategy, which are becoming more important for healthcare organizations. Additionally, key management functions, including finance, controlling, or a healthcare organizations' identity, can be significantly shaped by non-medical support services.

2.3. *Patient-centric and recovery-focused service provision*

As FM organizations improve their professionalization, they become more integrated with the core business (Ware *et al.*, 2017) and therefore increasingly interlink with other organizational functions (Nor *et al.*, 2014). The implementation of FM services can directly contribute to the advancement of the core business by enhancing workplace satisfaction and, in certain instances, even client productivity (Bröchner, 2017; Nutt, 1999; Van Sprang & Drion, 2020). In the healthcare setting, this is, for example, expressed through a holistic, interdisciplinary, and patient-centric approach toward a recovery-focused service provision, whereby the customer or patient's view lies at the core (*Gerber, 2021; Gerber et al.,* 2020). In this context, FM contributes to the delivery of high-quality hospitality services, offering friendly and positive guest interactions, hotel-like service standards, enjoyable and nutritious meals, superior hygiene, and clean environments among others. All of these aspects have a direct impact on patient and customer experience and perception.

3. The Digitalization of Healthcare Facility Management Services

The transition toward an interdisciplinary and patient-centric understanding of FM services described above is further underpinned by digital transformation. The often prevailing "silo mentality" of the disparate core and support services is no longer viable. Figure 2 outlines the digital transformation approach from the FM perspective. It is thereby important to recognize how the provision of FM services (as part of non-medical services) is an intersection between digital health and digital FM. To effectively realize such an integration of digital processes on the health and support service side, a cohesive collaboration among all stakeholders is required.

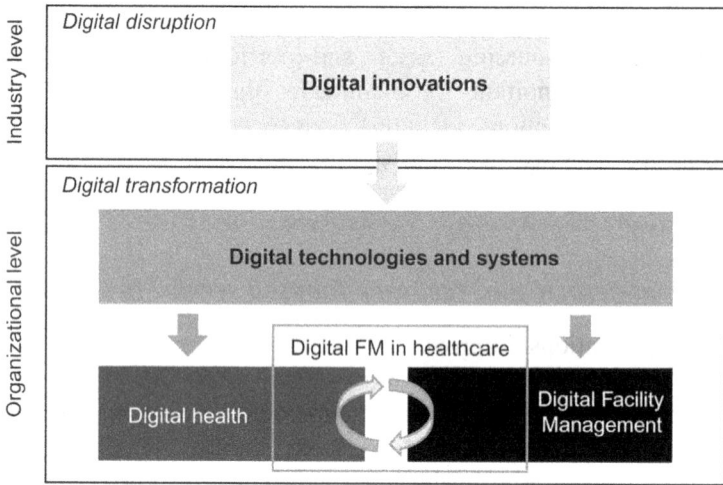

Figure 2.   Context and interrelation of digital FM in healthcare.

FM, with its horizontal logic, has the potential to play a crucial role in bridging the gap between the different disciplines (Lok *et al.*, 2023) which is necessary to realize a patient-centric digitalized service provision. To ensure a seamless delivery of healthcare services, the responsible digitalization teams must consider the specific adaptations required to deliver both the product and service optimally in a digitally enabled environment. To develop such integrated and unified solutions, the potential of all relevant technologies must be exploited. If FM aims to assume a leading role in this area, it must understand the advancements in digital FM as well as digital health. The following two sections provide an overview of both areas and their key technologies.

3.1. *Digital health*

Kostkova (2015) defines digital health as the "use of information and communications technologies to improve human health, healthcare services, and wellness for individuals and across populations" (p. 1). Key digital technologies which are used in digital health applications include artificial intelligence (AI), Internet of Things (IoT), big data, cyber physical systems (CPS), cloud computing (Tortorella *et al.*, 2020), robotics, smart logistics, wearable technologies, mobile applications, blockchain/ digital ledger technology (DLT), 3D printing, virtual assistants (VAs), 5G, augmented reality (AR)/virtual reality (VR), and digital twins (DTs) (Lee *et al.*, 2022). Pousttchi *et al.* (2019) characterize several key properties that define such digital technologies, which can be helpful when thinking about the attributes of digital health services (p. 487):

- large-scale and ubiquitous data processing,
- utilization of advanced machine learning (ML) techniques,
- extensive networking and communication,
- implementation of sophisticated human–computer interactions.

To further understand possible digital health domains, in which FM could be impacted or involved, the classification fields by Angerer and Berger (2023), as shown in Figure 3, are useful. These include the four quadrants: trend health, e-health, tech health, and data health. For FM, especially the dimensions tech health and data health are relevant. Although within the other two dimensions, there are application scenarios which have implications for FM. Tech health centers primarily on the hardware side of digital health applications, with particular focus on robotics and sensors. Though applications can be defined more broadly to include patient logistics, cleaning, or transportation of goods (Kolpashchikov *et al.*, 2022). With data health, solutions concerned with data generation,

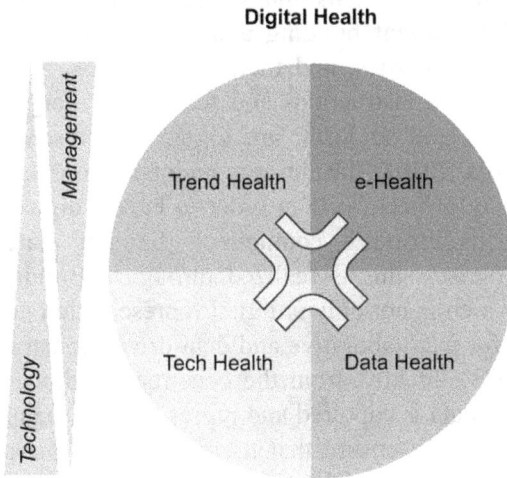

Figure 3. Classification of digital health fields.

Source: Adapted from *Der Digital Health Report 2023/2024: Mehr Digitalisierung im Gesundheitswesen wagen!* by Angerer and Berger (2023, p. 6).

management, and processing are central, including the main technologies of big data, IoT, and AI. These solutions often rely on data from other digital health applications and are therefore closely linked to them. Likewise, FM-relevant data, as, for example, from interior environments, can be tied into patient recovery evaluations (Nikabadi *et al.*, 2022).

Within digital health, many Ambient Assisted Living (AAL) products and services can be found, with certain smart home applications. AAL solutions combine a wide range of technologies to support older adults to live independently at home and are increasingly introduced into professional settings, such as elderly care homes and neighborhood development projects (Kofler *et al.*, 2019).

3.2. *Digital FM*

In spite of the relevance of digital health, FM applications remain at the heart of digitization efforts. The FM use cases in the healthcare sector are not particularly unlike those in other industries. However, the complexity is often greater and the stakes higher. Operational and supply interruptions to critical infrastructures, in particular, can have serious consequences. This increases the requirements baseline.

The concept of Common Data Environments (CDEs) is a fundamental technology that underpins many digitization efforts in the built environment. All relevant building and process information related to building entities, properties, and their relationships, as well as service systems, maintenance instructions and schedules, energy consumptions, indoor conditions, and so forth, are digitally represented in a central system (Halmetoja, 2019). The aim is to maintain this data repository over the entire building project cycle in order to have a digital representation of the building, its attributes, components, building materials, and processes. In most cases, this is realized through a Building Information Model (BIM) which is not only a digital representation and tool but also a methodology for a collaborative and data-driven construction approach (Borkowski, 2023). Ideally, from the construction process onwards, all relevant building data is captured and represented in the model. It is then especially important to ensure that the data from construction is transferred to operation (Ashworth and Tucker, 2021) because the information is vital for subsequent building life-cycle phases (Demirdöğen *et al.*, 2021). Many of the other digital technologies in FM build upon BIM (or a CDE), as is highlighted by Schmitter and Ashworth (2023).

To achieve the full potential though, it requires linking BIM with real-time data. In this case, the BIM model acts as a DT (Krämer *et al.*, 2022). To realize this, interconnected devices and sensors to collect data, a network layer to connect the devices, and a data management system are needed (Chen *et al.*, 2023). Real-time context data from the IoT environment is fused with the BIM model that represents the semantic relationships between building components (Huang *et al.*, 2023). With this dynamic and data-enriched BIM representation, facility managers have direct feedback on interventions, leading to continuous improvement of assets, services, and processes. To handle and make sense of the data advances, statistical analysis and ML algorithms are used. With predictive analytics, actionable information for detecting possible future equipment failures is possible (Olsen, 2020). With condition-based maintenance practices using IoT, more sustainable and cost-effective building services are possible.

The integration of physical objects through sensors, actuators, and software (Godager *et al.*, 2021) enables the collection and exchange of asset data. Core technologies such as radio frequency identification (RFID), location detection technologies (LDT), near-field communication (NFC), Bluetooth Low Energy (BLE), and Zigbee form the backbone of many of the IoT systems (Schmitter & Ashworth, 2023). These systems allow for different indoor positioning and navigation (IPIN) applications. By deploying sensor-based occupancy monitoring, dynamic representations of building usage are possible (Godager *et al.*, 2021), location-based services can be provided (Halmetoja, 2019), or location data that is critical during emergency situations can be accessed (Dahanayake and Sumanarathna, 2022). Other technologies, including AR and VR, offer novel interfaces, with which the user and Facility Managers can interact with digital content. For example, FM can collaborate with stakeholders on 3D BIM models of hospitals using AR or VR (Støre-Valen, 2021) to create immersive experiences for them to better visualize the spatial conditions for their processes.

As in many other areas of healthcare and in industries overall, AI has become one of the key technologies. AI has the potential to change FM services through "efficiency, scalability, reliability and predictability" (Zaki, 2019, p. 430). As an example, much of the unstructured data that forms CDEs can be efficiently tapped into through text mining (Santos *et al.*, 2023). State-of-the-art large language models (LLMs) have enabled the development of chatbot applications that introduce novel user interfaces and process automation. Chatbots can assist patients or healthcare staff in controlling room automation and appliances (Valtolina *et al.*, 2020). As already mentioned above, ML can be used to automate and optimize critical functions, such as energy management, heating, ventilation, and air conditioning (HVAC) control, or security monitoring (Viriato, 2019). ML is also used for Supply Chain Management (SCM) strategies to help improve forecasting of inventory, based on demand and supply (Gupta *et al.*, 2022). A further domain that is finding increased traction is robotics. For example, transport robots are used in healthcare to autonomously transfer items, such as medical supplies between hospital units (Holland *et al.*, 2021; Morgan *et al.*, 2022). Holland *et al.* (2021) further present how ultraviolet (UVC) light disinfection robots are deployed to autonomously navigate hospital rooms and eliminate micro-organisms. Other types of robots are used to clean and decontaminate surfaces and walls or high-touch points, such as doorknobs and tables.

The above examples represent an illustrative, though not exhaustive, selection of potential technologies and use cases. These examples demonstrate how (some emerging) digital technologies can potentially reshape FM processes, workflows, and services. Despite lower levels of automation in healthcare, there is clear potential for rapid adoption of these technologies, which will see more advanced solutions introduced.

4. Digital Transformation in FM in Healthcare

The two previous sections on digital health and digital FM introduced the various technologies that are driving digitalization in FM in healthcare. Rather than examining these technologies in isolation, the real challenge lies in their effective combination and integration into the complex socio-technical systems that characterize healthcare organizations. This demands a different mindset which embraces digital transformation as more than just a set of isolated digital solutions.

As highlighted by the European Union (2019) report on digital transformation of healthcare services, digitalization is less about the technological aspect and much more about being an "organisational and cultural process" (p. 13). For FM to succeed, digital technologies must be interwoven with their business logic and core operations, making them an integral and strategic part of the organizational unit. The literature often misinterprets digital transformation in FM as merely the adoption of

Digital Transformation Factors

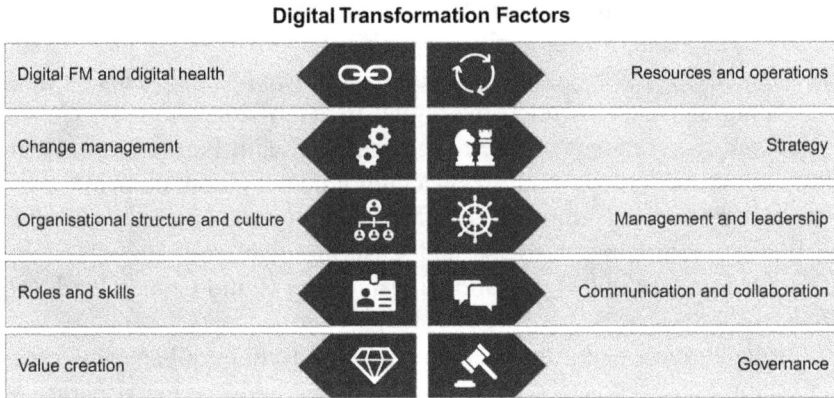

Figure 4. Digital transformation dimensions.

information technology (IT) solutions and data-driven processes. For instance, Atta and Talamo (2020) emphasize IoT and big data for enhancing maintenance, while Dahanayake and Sumanarathna (2022) point to IoT-BIM integration without exploring its broader implications. Pedral Sampaio *et al.* (2023) describe the digital transformation as a "digital transition", focusing on technologies such as BIM, AI, and IoT to optimize the building management of hospitals. Yet, all these perspectives tend to miss the mark when it comes to understanding digital transformation as an organizational capability.

This section therefore aims to broaden the technological focus by providing a holistic view of digital transformation for healthcare FM services. This chapter introduces 10 dimensions (shown in Figure 4) to provide FM leaders with a broader perspective. Each of these dimensions is elaborated in more detail to provide the necessary knowledge and tools to think strategically about digital transformation.

4.1. *Change management*

Facility Managers should pay close attention when considering taking a proactive approach toward change management. Too often, it becomes a point of failure because it is not given sufficient scrutiny (Correani *et al.*, 2020). The question is how to set up the organization to optimally implement and leverage new digital technologies (Fung-Kee-Fung and Michalowski, 2019). In principle, with a top-down approach, the entire healthcare organization undergoes a (continuous) change process. For Facility Managers, it is crucial to be actively involved in the process and act as ambassadors for the change within their own FM unit. This requires translating and implementing the digital transformation strategy, change vision and requirements for their organizational unit. Furthermore, attention should be laid on mobilizing commitment by communicating the vision, empowering employees, effectively promoting skills and role adaptation, removing barriers, and ensuring that new processes are embedded under the FM operational framework (Pulido and Taherdoost, 2023).

Collaboration with other departments and forming alliances is especially important, given the cross-organizational and horizontal nature of FM. These partnerships can span a wide range of domains, including skills training and pooling, the implementation of learning and development systems, and effectively managing the change process (Fung-Kee-Fung and Michalowski, 2019). This task is very complex and correspondingly challenging, especially in healthcare organizations, which are often hierarchical and organized in silos with highly specialized fields.

If the overall organization is not yet ready for the digital transformation, FM can build up its change readiness to lay the foundation for the future change process (Armenakis *et al.*, 1993). Managers can already act as a change agent, priming the organizational unit for digital transformation by reducing resistance and influencing mindsets.

4.2. *Organizational structure and culture*

Facility Managers must also consider adapting existing FM and organizational structures in the context of the digital transformation. Primary reasons for restructuring are to enhance collaboration within and across the organization, improve transparency, achieve operational standardization, increase efficiency, and eliminate silo-thinking and fragmentation (Cennamo *et al.*, 2020; Westerman *et al.*, 2014). Typically, a digital transformation leads to a closer alignment of business units (Ekman *et al.*, 2019), as they become increasingly interwoven through digital processes. This necessitates that FM aligns its services, processes, and strategies to support these integrated efforts as part of its organizational restructuring.

The literature on digital transformation often references the formation of a centralized transformation or innovation unit (see Chaniot (2019),

Fischer (2020), and Westerman (2014)). Guinan *et al.* (2019) described this central unit as "digital hub", which can facilitate the organization of resources, training, support, etc. throughout the entire organization. It is advisable for FM to be part of any such initiative, proactively shaping and promoting the transformation while also benefiting from cross-organizational exchange. In addition to the centralized digital hub, individual organizational units must retain the ability to execute the digital transformation under their own authority. This offers FM organizations the opportunity to steer their own transformation and potentially emerge as digital leaders, setting best practices for the entire healthcare organization.

Though, to become leaders of a digital transformation, FM needs to focus on cultivating an appropriate organizational culture. Culture is recognized as a key lever for the success of any digital transformation (Firican, 2024; Martínez-Caro *et al.*, 2020; Rautenbach *et al.*, 2019) and can be seen as an extension of the transformation strategy. A digital mindset is characterized by openness to risk-taking, experimentation, ideation, and learning in a digital setting (Rowles and Brown, 2017). FM leaders should encourage and communicate this mindset to foster behaviors that support innovation where possible. Firican (2024), for example, provides a comprehensive overview and practical actions based on a literature review of digital culture, encompassing 13 dimensions that can guide successful transformation initiatives.

4.3. Roles and skills

With changes in organizational structure and culture, new roles and skills need to follow. It is those skills, capabilities, and new roles that are fundamental drivers of digital transformation (Brock and Wangenheim, 2019; Varian, 2018). While traditional competencies in FM, such as those, for example, defined by IFMA (2022), remain crucial, they must now be complemented by skills that support the digital transformation. Table 1 offers an overview of these emerging requirements, as found in the digital transformation literature. The comparisons of the digital transformation skill requirements with the FM core competencies show that facility information management, technology management, leadership and strategy, communication, performance and quality, as well as project management are most likely areas that will become more important.

Table 1. Skill requirements for the digital transformation.

Skill category	Skills	Description
Strategic management	Vision	Long-term, big-picture planning
	Shared understanding	Ensuring alignment across teams
Tactical management	Coordination	Managing interdependent activities
	Cross-collaboration	Encouraging collaboration across departments
	Troubleshooting	Solving technical and operational issues
Information and technology	Data management	Organizing and securing data for operational insights
	Analytics	Analyzing data to drive decisions
	Programming	Development of software/tools to support digital initiatives and processes
	Application development	Creating applications for FM operations
	Security	Ensuring digital safety and compliance
	Cross-channel integration	Linking systems across platforms for seamless interaction
Interpersonal/soft skills	Communication	Facilitating clear and consistent messaging across appropriate channels
	Collaboration	Encouraging teamwork and shared goals
	Teamwork	Building unified approach among staff

Source: Information based on Berman (2012); Guinan *et al.* (2019); Kazim (2019); McAfee and Brynjolfsson (2017); Rowles and Brown (2017).

Defining roles and skills across all organizational units, as suggested by Correani *et al.* (2020), helps avoid redundancies and streamline training and hiring. Based on this, the roles and skills of FM can be derived and aligned. Once the skill requirements are defined, FM leaders must determine the optimal skill-grade mix for their organization. Necessary skills can either be acquired from outside or built up internally. This should be at the forefront of facility managers' thinking when developing their digital transformation capabilities. One of FM's strengths as a generalist discipline, with its horizontal management focus, is that it can more likely build up and cultivate so-called "T-shaped employees" – those with deep technical or domain-specific expertise, combined with broad interpersonal skills and an overview of the entire operational procedures (Guinan *et al.*, 2019). In this way, it is foreseeable that FM can thrive in a digital transformation, as it can bridge functional gaps while strategically driving digital initiatives.

4.4. *Value creation*

Rather than focusing solely on technology functions, FM leaders must also prioritize value creation. This shift in perspective should be at the forefront of every strategic discussion. In much of the business management literature on digital transformation, the primary goal described is to increase customer value (Furjan *et al.*, 2020; Mammen, 2022; Shaughnessy, 2018; Westerman *et al.*, 2014). In healthcare organizations, emphasis is especially given to improving patient recovery outcomes. For FM, this means thinking about how digital technologies can potentially enhance its services and the built environment to improve, directly or indirectly, a patient's recovery process. Value can also be created for visitors or internal employees. To further illustrate how value can be created in facility service areas, consider the following examples:

- *Hospitality services*: Improving accommodation management through better patient interaction technologies.
- *Catering and food services*: Utilizing machine vision to monitor food and nutrient consumption, allowing for improved custom meal planning that aligns with patient or resident preferences and dietary needs.
- *Safety and security*: Implementing comprehensive fall detection sensors throughout the premises and integrating them with staff management systems to grant more autonomy to residents.
- *Accommodation management and operation of properties*: Leveraging IPIN technology to assist relatives accompanying patients in navigating the building.

Value can be framed in terms of safety, convenience, quality, information, or comfort for patients, visitors, and staff. To assess and strategize value creation, FM leaders can make use of available frameworks, including value mapping by Green and Jack (2004), Vischer's (2005) habitability pyramid, Bitner's (1992) environment–user relationships, or the relationship value framework by Cui and Coenen (2016). Also, Gerber's (2021) recovery-focused service provision concept provides a useful lens for understanding value creation for patients.

Generating added value involves reconfiguring processes and fostering new collaborations, often requiring a networked approach. Creating and delivering value increasingly depends on collaborating with multiple stakeholders. That is why it is advantageous to develop digital business models (BMs). Digital BMs serve as strategic instruments that guide how technology can be embedded into the business logic or ecosystem – helping define relationships, resource processes, and value creation. The BM lies at the intersection of strategy and business operations (Osterwalder *et al.*, 2005) and further reinforces the digital transformation.

4.5. Resources and operations

Resources play a crucial yet tacit role in leveraging digital technologies across an organization. Effective resource management must be a strategic issue for digital transformation (Clifton *et al.*, 2020; Koch *et al.*, 2019). Healthcare organizations frequently struggle with resources while implementing digital applications, often due to unclear coordination of processes. A strategic approach, as suggested by Guenzi and Habel (2020), involves mapping out all processes. Process architectures serve as valuable tools for assessing the current status and planning transformation efforts. Initial focus should be on "low-hanging fruit," initiatives requiring minimal effort, yet yielding high impact. In this context, it is important for FM and IT to work closely together, as IT resources are often limited, and multiple IT-related implementation projects may run concurrently. Prioritizing and bundling projects helps prevent redundant applications. For example, a procurement system for medical products could also be adapted for non-medical consumables.

A digital mindset proves beneficial for digital operations, requiring rapid integration of new developments, agile problem-solving (Guinan *et al.*, 2019), and reducing barriers between stakeholders (Correani *et al.*, 2020).

Organizations that adopt a learning approach, open to experimentation and collaboration, are generally more successful in their digital transformation initiatives (Guinan *et al.*, 2019). Once implemented, Kretschmer and Khashabi (2020) found that a digital transformation can significantly impact internal processes, providing more information for grouping tasks, enhancing skill requirements, matching tasks with agents, and improving task completion through monitoring and analytics.

4.6. *Strategy*

A well-defined strategy is essential and a prerequisite for successful digital transformation. As discussed earlier, digital BMs then bridge the gap between strategy and operational levels, facilitating effective value delivery. The digital transformation strategy must align with the overall organizational strategy (e.g., a hospital strategy) while fully exploiting the benefits of digitalization. It should not only adapt the organizational strategy but also create a clear awareness of the digital transformation itself (Sandkuhl *et al.*, 2019). It provides a clear direction, highlighting priorities and ensuring alignment between organizational units. In essence, the strategy governs the overall transformation process (Cosa, 2024). Leaders need to articulate the purpose of transformation clearly, defining both the opportunities and challenges, as well as setting clear business outcomes (Lawson and Weberg, 2023).

As a prerequisite, an in-depth analysis of the health policy landscape, market trends, competitor strategies, etc. is crucial. Moreover, it is also advisable to assess the digital maturity of the healthcare organization (Kirecci *et al.*, 2022). Once a foundational business analysis is performed, the transformation intent can be clarified. A compelling vision is also integral to the strategy. Westerman *et al.* (2014) suggest the vision should be transformative, focused on intent and outcome, reflect the organization's strengths, align with core skills, and endorse the novel recombination of digital and physical assets.

To ensure successful implementation, key stakeholders must be involved in the strategy development process (Graf *et al.*, 2019). The strategy should reflect the organization's unique context and encompass all relevant medical and non-medical areas, which is why FM must be involved in the strategy formulation process from the beginning. FM leaders then must translate the transformation strategy into a functional-level, (digital) FM strategy, distinct from the overarching business strategy but aligned to contribute to strategic goals (see Chen *et al.*, (2010)). It needs to be kept in mind that the adoption of a digital transformation strategy requires constant negotiation and flexibility, as it is not always a linear process (Ekman *et al.*, 2019). Facility managers need to embrace the idea that the entire process involves collaboration with various stakeholders through ongoing reviews to ensure alignment and success.

4.7. *Management and leadership*

Strong leadership from senior management (including FM) is crucial for a successful digital transformation, particularly to guide the organization through this complex process (Rakovic *et al.*, 2024). Management is responsible for building and developing the organizational capabilities necessary for effective transformation (Gfrerer *et al.*, 2021). However, clarity is needed about who leads the transformation at both strategic and FM levels. Some organizations appoint a Chief Digital Officer (CDO) to promote the digital transformation at an executive level (Chaniot, 2019; Rowles and Brown, 2017). Nevertheless, a "buy in" from senior management is essential.

Middle management, such as Facility Managers, also plays a key role in leading and managing the transformation on tactical and operational levels. Middle managers are often under significant pressure to implement digital changes and lead employees through the transition (Guinan *et al.*, 2019). Therefore, FM leaders must ensure that adequate resources and support are provided. Facility managers can utilize various tools to drive digital transformation. These include building a coalition of supporters, crowdsourcing ideas from employees, fostering open communication, and leveraging internal information for decision-making (Westerman *et al.*, 2014). Using key performance indicators (KPIs) can also help in communicating and measuring the progress of transformation efforts.

Facility managers may become advocates for digital transformation. This requires digital leadership, which embodies strong beliefs in success, resilience, continuous learning, and confidence in digitalization efforts, among others (April and Dalwai, 2019; Tigre *et al.*, 2024). In this regard, Tigre *et al.* (2024) provide a comprehensive overview and conceptual model of digital leadership capabilities.

4.8. *Communication and collaboration*

Communication touches nearly every level of digital transformation. It is crucial in empowering employees, promoting new roles, and ensuring effective collaboration. For Facility Managers, communication is particularly important, as they work with diverse groups of employees, from cleaning staff and building technicians to health and safety managers, across operational, tactical, and strategic levels. They must therefore adapt their messaging to suit different stakeholders. It is vital that information is conveyed in a way that is understandable, transparent, and applicable to each group (Westerman *et al.*, 2014). Moreover, it is necessary to determine the appropriate digital channels and frequency for communication. The digital transformation entails that FM leaders must engage more frequently with a wide range of stakeholders, making effective communication even more relevant.

Digital projects often involve multidisciplinary and cross-functional teams. Dugstad *et al.* (2019), in their case study on the introduction of digital monitoring systems in nursing homes, stress the importance of co-creation across professional and organizational boundaries. Similarly, Barnett *et al.* (2019) found that multidisciplinary teams in healthcare often included a range of skills, from clinical owners to data analysts and end-user clinicians. Collaboration works on multiple levels, involving business, technical, and functional specialists (April and Dalwai, 2019). Facility Managers need to be aware of this and adapt communication to ensure that all team members, regardless of their discipline or function, are aligned and informed throughout the transformation process.

4.9. *Governance*

Whereas the digital transformation strategy, vision, and digital mindset give a certain freedom and openness to experimentation, governance sets guardrails for what is feasible and what is not. This is particularly crucial in healthcare organizations, where sensitive data and high ethical standards are involved. However, overly stringent governance can stifle digital transformation. The goal of governance in digital transformation is to set clear rules and responsibilities, frame the implementation process (Westerman *et al.*, 2014), and establish appropriate control mechanisms

(Fischer *et al.*, 2020). Thus, existing corporate governance models often need to be adapted to accommodate the digital transformation (Dicuonzo *et al.*, 2023).

In this process, FM should play a role in finding the right balance between different interests, strategies, and positions to be effective with their digitalization of FM services (April and Dalwai, 2019; Rowles and Brown, 2017). April and Dalwai (2019) emphasize that without a push to adapt governance modes to favor digital transformation, governance elements may become obstacles. Compared to the medical sector, non-medical areas often present fewer data protection risks, allowing for easier implementation of digital solutions. Therefore, early and proactive intervention to promote digitalization and adopt governance requirements is important.

5. Discussion and Conclusion

The rather constrained traditional approach to the digital transformation of healthcare FM services is clearly not sufficient. The digital transformation is multidimensional and extends on a technological level from dedicated digital FM solutions to the broad spectrum of digital health applications. The list of digital technologies from both domains highlights the sheer number of possibilities for designing services around them. This underscores the necessity for healthcare providers to place greater emphasis on actually developing new services around these digital technologies. Therefore, decision-makers have to consider more about the integration and combination of multiple technologies, the proliferation and embeddedness of them, and the use of data processing while designing new digital health service solutions. Moreover, the ongoing evolution of digital systems is leading toward greater automation, which opens up entirely new possibilities for processes. Traditional siloed process designs are not sufficient in this respect. A fundamental shift in perspective and awareness is required with regard to digital transformation. To this end, digital technologies must be embedded throughout processes, requiring a multiperspective approach to the design of high-quality, patient-centric services.

As a strategic organizational unit, FM is clearly a crucial player in the digital transformation. This necessitates though, that Facility Managers adopt a more expansive, strategic, and holistic approach, as presented by the 10 digital transformation dimensions. Nine of those aim at organizational fundamentals, such as culture, structure, value creation, strategy, or leadership. It is argued here that this approach can significantly increase

the impact of FM digitization efforts. Given the extent of services provided, the service-oriented perspective, the relationships across functional
units, and the impact of the built environment on the entire healthcare
organization, FM can make a significant contribution. The key to this lies
in the hands of FM leaders who recognize the relevance and have the
necessary knowledge of the strategic levers of digital transformation.

References

Angerer, A. and Berger, S. (2023). *Der Digital Health Report 2023/2024:
Mehr Digitalisierung im Gesundheitswesen wagen!* MWV Medizinisch
Wissenschaftliche Verlagsgesellschaft.

April, K. and Dalwai, A. (2019). Leadership styles required to lead digital
transformation. *Effective Executive*, *22*(2), 14–45.

Armenakis, A. A., Harris, S. G., and Mossholder, K. W. (1993). Creating
readiness for organizational change. *Human Relations*, *46*(6), 681–703.

Ashworth, S. and Tucker, M. (2021). *FM-BIM Mobilisation Framework: Critical
Success Factors to Help Deliver Successful BIM Projects* [118, application/
pdf]. Liverpool John Moores University. https://doi.org/10.21256/ZHAW-
24021.

Atta, N. and Talamo, C. (2020). Digital transformation in facility management
(FM). IoT and big data for service innovation. In B. Daniotti, M. Gianinetto,
and S. Della Torre (Eds.), *Digital Transformation of the Design, Construction
and Management Processes of the Built Environment*, pp. 267–278. Springer
International Publishing.

Barnett, A., Winning, M., Canaris, S., Cleary, M., Staib, A., and Sullivan, C.
(2019). Digital transformation of hospital quality and safety: Real-time data
for real-time action. *Australian Health Review*, *43*(6), 656.

Berman, S. J. (2012). Digital transformation: Opportunities to create new
business models. *Strategy & Leadership*, *40*(2), 16–24.

Bitner, M. J. (1992). Servicescapes: The impact of physical surroundings on
customers and employees. *Journal of Marketing*, *56*(2), 57–71.

Borkowski, A. S. (2023). A literature review of BIM definitions: Narrow and
broad views. *Technologies*, *11*(6), 176.

Bröchner, J. (2017). Measuring the productivity of facilities management.
Journal of Facilities Management, *15*(3), 285–301.

Cennamo, C., Dagnino, G. B., Di Minin, A., and Lanzolla, G. (2020). Managing
digital transformation: Scope of transformation and modalities of value
co-generation and delivery. *California Management Review*, *62*(4), 5–16.

Chaniot, E. (2019). Tools for transformation: Michelin's digital journey.
Research-Technology Management, *62*(6), 31–35.

Chen, D. Q., Mocker, M., Preston, D. S., and Teubner, A. (2010). Information systems strategy: Reconceptualization, measurement, and implications. *MIS Quarterly, 34*(2), 233.

Chen, Y., Wang, X., Liu, Z., Cui, J., Osmani, M., and Demian, P. (2023). Exploring building information modeling (BIM) and internet of things (IoT) integration for sustainable building. *Buildings, 13*(2), 288.

Clifton, J., Díaz Fuentes, D., and Llamosas García, G. (2020). ICT-enabled co-production of public services: Barriers and enablers. A systematic review. *Information Polity, 25*(1), 25–48.

Coenen, C. and Von Felten, D. (2014). A service-oriented perspective of facility management. *Facilities, 32*(9/10), 554–564.

Correani, A., De Massis, A., Frattini, F., Petruzzelli, A. M., and Natalicchio, A. (2020). Implementing a digital strategy: Learning from the experience of three digital transformation projects. *California Management Review, 62*(4), 37–56.

Cosa, M. (2024). Business digital transformation: Strategy adaptation, communication and future agenda. *Journal of Strategy and Management, 17*(2), 244–259.

Cui, Y. Y. and Coenen, C. (2016). Relationship value in outsourced FM services – value dimensions and drivers. *Facilities, 34*(1/2), 43–68.

Dahanayake, K. C. and Sumanarathna, N. (2022). IoT-BIM-based digital transformation in facilities management: A conceptual model. *Journal of Facilities Management, 20*(3), 437–451.

Demirdöğen, G., Diren, N. S., Aladağ, H., and Işık, Z. (2021). Lean based maturity framework integrating value, BIM and big data analytics: Evidence from AEC industry. *Sustainability, 13*(18), 10029.

Dicuonzo, G., Donofrio, F., Fusco, A., and Shini, M. (2023). Healthcare system: Moving forward with artificial intelligence. *Technovation, 120*, 102510.

Dugstad, J., Eide, T., Nilsen, E. R., and Eide, H. (2019). Towards successful digital transformation through co-creation: A longitudinal study of a four-year implementation of digital monitoring technology in residential care for persons with dementia. *BMC Health Services Research, 19*(1), 366.

Ekman, P., Thilenius, P., Thompson, S., and Whitaker, J. (2019). Digital transformation of global business processes: The role of dual embeddedness. *Business Process Management Journal, 26*(2), 570–592.

European Union (2019). *Assessing the Impact of Digital Transformation of Health Services: Report of the Expert Panel on Effective Ways of Investing in Health (EXPH).* Publications Office of the European Union. https://doi.org/10.2875/644722.

Firican, D. A. (2024). Creating a digital culture for digital transformation: A literature review of practical steps. *Proceedings of the International Conference on Business Excellence, 18*(1), 1018–1028.

Fischer, M., Imgrund, F., Janiesch, C., and Winkelmann, A. (2020). Strategy archetypes for digital transformation: Defining meta objectives using business process management. *Information & Management*, *57*(5), 103262.

Fung-Kee-Fung, M. and Michalowski, W. (2019). Business school teams up with clinical innovators: An opportunity for health system transformation. *Healthcare Management Forum*, *32*(4), 218–223.

Furjan, M. T., Tomičić-Pupek, K., and Pihir, I. (2020). Understanding digital transformation initiatives: Case studies analysis. *Business Systems Research Journal*, *11*(1), 125–141.

Gerber, N. (2021). *Model for a Holistic, Interdisciplinary and Interprofessional Recovery-Focussed Service Provision in Health Organisations*. Working Paper of the Institute for Facility Management, ZHAW Zürcher Hochschule für Angewandte Wissenschaften. https://digitalcollection.zhaw.ch/handle/11475/22581.

Gerber, N., Kirecci, I., Klauser, V., Krähenbühl, A., Nörr-Pfenninger, S., Pericin Häfliger, I., Schmitter, P., and Hofer, S. (2020). *Service- und genesungsorientierte Leistungserstellung in Gesundheitsorganisationen: Ein Plädoyer für mehr Kooperation von medizinischen und nicht-medizinischen Berufsgruppen*. Working Paper of the Institute for Facility Management, ZHAW Zürcher Hochschule für Angewandte Wissenschaften. https://digitalcollection.zhaw.ch/handle/11475/21153.

Gerber, N. and Kuchen, O. (2019). *Service Catalogue for Non-Medical Services in Hospitals (LekaS): Version 2.0: Translation of the German Original*. ZHAW Zürcher Hochschule für Angewandte Wissenschaften. https://digitalcollection.zhaw.ch/handle/11475/19151.

Gfrerer, A., Hutter, K., Füller, J., and Ströhle, T. (2021). Ready or not: Managers' and employees' different perceptions of digital readiness. *California Management Review*, *63*(2), 23–48.

Godager, B., Onstein, E., and Huang, L. (2021). The concept of enterprise BIM: Current research practice and future trends. *IEEE Access*, *9*, 42265–42290.

Graf, M., Peter, M., and Gatziu-Grivas, S. (2019). Foster strategic orientation in the digital age: A methodic approach for guiding SME to a digital transformation. In W. Abramowicz and A. Paschke (Eds.), *Business Information Systems Workshops*, Vol. 339, pp. 420–432. Springer International Publishing.

Green, A. N. and Jack, A. (2004). Creating stakeholder value by consistently aligning the support environment with stakeholder needs. *Facilities*, *22*(13/14), 359–363.

Guenzi, P. and Habel, J. (2020). Mastering the digital transformation of sales. *California Management Review*, *62*(4), 57–85.

Guinan, P. J., Parise, S., and Langowitz, N. (2019). Creating an innovative digital project team: Levers to enable digital transformation. *Business Horizons*, *62*(6), 717–727.

Gupta, A. K., Awatade, G. V., Padole, S. S., and Choudhari, Y. S. (2022). Digital supply chain management using AI, ML and blockchain. In K. Perumal, C. L. Chowdhary, and L. Chella (Eds.), *Innovative Supply Chain Management via Digitalization and Artificial Intelligence*, Vol. 424, pp. 1–19. Springer, Singapore.

Hakimi, O., Liu, H., and Abudayyeh, O. (2024). Digital twin-enabled smart facility management: A bibliometric review. *Frontiers of Engineering Management, 11*(1), 32–49.

Halmetoja, E. (2019). The conditions data model supporting building information models in facility management. *Facilities, 37*(7/8), 484–501.

Hofer, S. and Gerber, N. (2015). Role model for chief facility managing officers (CFMOs) based on the service allocation model for service companies (SAMoS): A theoretical reflection and basis for discussion. *EuroFM Research Papers 2015, EuroFM 2015 Proceedings.* https://doi.org/10.21256/zhaw-1488.

Holland, J., Kingston, L., McCarthy, C., Armstrong, E., O'Dwyer, P., Merz, F., and McConnell, M. (2021). Service robots in the healthcare sector. *Robotics, 10*(1), 47.

Huang, X., Liu, Y., Huang, L., Onstein, E., and Merschbrock, C. (2023). BIM and IoT data fusion: The data process model perspective. *Automation in Construction, 149*, 104792.

Huynh, D. and Nguyen-Ky, S. (2020). Engaging building automation data visualisation using building information modelling and progressive web application. *Open Engineering, 10*(1), 434–442.

IFMA (2022). 11 core competencies of facility management. *Knowledge Library*, January. https://knowledgelibrary.ifma.org/11-core-competencies-of-facility-management/.

International Organization for Standardization (2017). *Facility management—Vocabulary* (No. ISO Standard No. 41011:2017). https://www.iso.org/standard/68167.html.

Kazim, F. (2019). Digital transformation and leadership style: A multiple case study. *The ISM Journal of International Business, 3*(1), 24–33.

Kirecci, I., Schmitter, P., Hanne, T., Gachnang, P., and Gatziu Grivas, S. (2022). *Reifegradmodelle als Grundlage für den digitalen Veränderungsprozess im Facility Management in Healthcare – Eine integrative Literaturrecherche.* https://doi.org/10.34749/JFM.2022.4634.

Koch, C., Hansen, G. K., and Jacobsen, K. (2019). Missed opportunities: Two case studies of digitalization of FM in hospitals. *Facilities, 37*(7/8), 381–394.

Kofler, A., Schmitter, P., Brockes, C., and Hofer, S. (2019). Service innovation for new care landscapes: A case study on safety in senior living and care. In J. Smithwick, K. Sullivan, and M. Bown (Eds.), *ASFM Fall 2019 Colloquium*, pp. 9–16. ASFM - Associated schools of Facility Management Proceedings.

Kolpashchikov, D., Gerget, O., and Meshcheryakov, R. (2022). Robotics in healthcare. In C.-P. Lim, Y.-W. Chen, A. Vaidya, C. Mahorkar, and L. C. Jain (Eds.), *Handbook of Artificial Intelligence in Healthcare*, Vol. 212, pp. 281–306. Springer International Publishing.

Kostkova, P. (2015). Grand challenges in digital health. *Frontiers in Public Health, 3*.

Krämer, M., Bender, T., Bock, N., Härtig, M., Jaspers, E., Koch, S., Opić, M., and Schlundt, M. (2022). IT-Umgebungen für BIM im FM. In M. May, M. Krämer, and M. Schlundt (Eds.), *BIM im Immobilienbetrieb*, pp. 103–132. Springer Fachmedien Wiesbaden.

Kretschmer, T. and Khashabi, P. (2020). Digital transformation and organization design: An integrated approach. *California Management Review, 62*(4), 86–104.

Lavikka, R. H., Lehtinen, T., and Hall, D. (2017). Co-creating digital services with and for facilities management. *Facilities, 35*(9/10), 543–556.

Lavy, S. and Shohet, I. M. (2007). A strategic integrated healthcare facility management model. *International Journal of Strategic Property Management, 11*(3), 125–142.

Lavy, S. and Terzioğlu, S. (2023). Delivery of healthcare facility management services: A literature review. *IOP Conference Series: Earth and Environmental Science, 1176*(1), 012017.

Lawson, C. and Weberg, D. (2023). Leading through times of transformation: Purpose, trust, and co-creation. *Nurse Leader, 21*(3), 380–384.

Lee, K., Seo, L., Yoon, D., Yang, K., Yi, J.-E., Kim, Y., and Lee, J.-H. (2022). Digital health profile of South Korea: A cross sectional study. *International Journal of Environmental Research and Public Health, 19*(10), 6329.

Lennerts, K., Abel, J., Pfründer, U., and Sharma, V. (2003). Reducing health care costs through optimised facility management-related processes. *Journal of Facilities Management, 2*(2), 192–206.

Lerzynski, G. (2021). Opening the door for digital transformation in hospitals: Management's point of view. In P. Glauner, P. Plugmann, and G. Lerzynski (Eds.), *Digitalization in Healthcare*, pp. 17–28. Springer International Publishing.

Lok, K. L., Van Der Pool, I., Smith, A. J., Opoku, A., and Cheung, K. L. (2023). Sustainable digitalisation and implementation of ISO standards for facilities management. *Facilities, 41*(5/6), 434–453.

Mammen, A. (2022). The digital transformation of a metropolitan New York health system. *Frontiers of Health Services Management, 38*(3), 10–15.

Martínez-Caro, E., Cegarra-Navarro, J. G., and Alfonso-Ruiz, F. J. (2020). Digital technologies and firm performance: The role of digital organisational culture. *Technological Forecasting and Social Change, 154*, 119962.

McAfee, A. and Brynjolfsson, E. (2017). *Machine, Platform, Crowd: Harnessing Our Digital Future*, First Edition. W.W. Norton & Company.

Morgan, A. A., Abdi, J., Syed, M. A. Q., Kohen, G. E., Barlow, P., and Vizcaychipi, M. P. (2022). Robots in healthcare: A scoping review. *Current Robotics Reports*, *3*(4), 271–280.

Nikabadi, S., Zabihi, H., and Shahcheraghi, A. (2022). Evaluating the effective factors of hospital rooms on patients' recovery using the data mining method. *HERD: Health Environments Research & Design Journal*, *15*(1), 97–114.

Nutt, B. (1999). Linking FM practice and research. *Facilities*, *17*(1/2), 11–17.

Olsen, T. (2020). Understanding the digital transformation. *Chemical Engineering Progress*, *116*(9), 29–35.

Osterwalder, A., Pigneur, Y., and Tucci, C. L. (2005). Clarifying business models: Origins, present, and future of the concept. *Communications of the Association for Information Systems*, *16*.

Paliderova, M. and Michalikova, K. F. (2018). Theoretical background of facility management. In N. Tsounis and A. Vlachvei (Eds.), *Advances in Time Series Data Methods in Applied Economic Research*, pp. 503–509. Springer International Publishing.

Pedral Sampaio, R., Aguiar Costa, A., and Flores-Colen, I. (2023). A discussion of digital transition impact on facility management of hospital buildings. *Facilities*, *41*(5/6), 389–406.

Pousttchi, K., Gleiss, A., Buzzi, B., and Kohlhagen, M. (2019). Technology impact types for digital transformation. *2019 IEEE 21st Conference on Business Informatics (CBI)*, 487–494.

Pulido, F. L. P. and Taherdoost, H. (2023). Managing change in the digital age: A comparative study of change management and digital transformation models. *2023 4th International Conference on Electronics and Sustainable Communication Systems (ICESC)*, 983–989.

Rakovic, L., Maric, S., Djordjevic Milutinovic, L., Vukovic, V., and Bjekic, R. (2024). The role of leadership in managing digital transformation: A systematic literature review. *E+M Ekonomie a Management*, *27*(2), 87–107.

Rautenbach, W. J., Kock, I. D., and Jooste, J. L. (2019). The development of a conceptual model for enabling a value-adding digital transformation: A conceptual model that aids organisations in the digital transformation process. *2019 IEEE International Conference on Engineering, Technology and Innovation (ICE/ITMC)*, 1–10.

Redlein, A. and Höhenberger, C. (2020). Digitalisation. In A. Redlein (Ed.), *Modern Facility and Workplace Management*, pp. 139–175. Springer International Publishing.

Rowles, D. and Brown, T. (2017). *Building Digital Culture: A Practical Guide to Successful Digital Transformation*. Kogan Page.

Sampaio, R. P., Costa, A. A., and Flores-Colen, I. (2023). Discussion of digital transition impact on the facility management sector applied to healthcare buildings. *IOP Conference Series: Earth and Environmental Science*, *1176*(1), 012014.

Sandkuhl, K., Shilov, N., and Smirnov, A. (2019). Facilitating digital transformation by multi-aspect ontologies: Approach and application steps. *IFAC-PapersOnLine*, *52*(13), 1609–1614.

Santos, P., Datia, N., Pato, M., Sobral, J., Gomes, N., Leitão, N., and Ferreira, M. R. (2023). NLP for enterprise asset management: An emerging paradigm. *2023 27th International Conference Information Visualisation (IV)*, 238–243.

Schmitter, P. and Ashworth, S. (2023). Digitally transforming facility management in healthcare: A systematic review of key digital technologies and systems. *IOP Conference Series: Earth and Environmental Science*, *1176*(1), 012012.

Shaughnessy, H. (2018). Creating digital transformation: Strategies and steps. *Strategy & Leadership*, *46*(2), 19–25.

Støre-Valen, M. (2021). FM and clinical employees' involvement in the design of eight Norwegian hospital projects. *Facilities*, *39*(11/12), 778–801.

Tigre, F. B., Henriques, P. L., and Curado, C. (2024). The digital leadership emerging construct: A multi-method approach. *Management Review Quarterly*.

Tortorella, G. L., Fogliatto, F. S., Mac Cawley Vergara, A., Vassolo, R., and Sawhney, R. (2020). Healthcare 4.0: Trends, challenges and research directions. *Production Planning & Control*, *31*(15), 1245–1260.

Valtolina, S., Barricelli, B. R., and Di Gaetano, S. (2020). Communicability of traditional interfaces VS chatbots in healthcare and smart home domains. *Behaviour & Information Technology*, *39*(1), 108–132.

Van Sprang, H. and Drion, B. (2020). *Introduction to Facility Management*, 1st Edition. Routledge.

Viriato, J. C. (2019). AI and machine learning in real estate investment. *The Journal of Portfolio Management*, *45*(7), 43–54.

Vischer, J. (2005). *Space Meets Status: Designing Workplace Performance*. Routledge.

Wang, Y., Wang, X., Wang, J., Yung, P., and Jun, G. (2013). Engagement of facilities management in design stage through BIM: Framework and a case study. *Advances in Civil Engineering*, *2013*, 1–8.

Westerman, G., Bonnet, D., and McAfee, A. (2014). *Leading Digital: Turning Technology into Business Transformation*. Harvard Business Review Press.

Zaki, M. (2019). Digital transformation: Harnessing digital technologies for the next generation of services. *Journal of Services Marketing*, *33*(4), 429–435.

Chapter 6

The Simulation Century: Harnessing AI and Simulation to Design a Better Future: A Personal Perspective

Richard James Boyd

CEO, UltiSim, USA

1. Introduction

In 2007, when the aerospace giant Lockheed Martin acquired my computer game technology company 3Dsolve, I gained unique insights into how large organizations tackle complex challenges. Over the next five and a half years, I witnessed firsthand the limitations of traditional approaches to solving increasingly complex problems. Whether dealing with space travel, stealth fighter aircraft, autonomous systems, or cyber security, Lockheed applied its century-old methodology of centralized systems integration – an approach that proved both expensive and time-consuming.

As Director of Emerging and Disruptive Technologies, I recognized the need to accelerate innovation by building on the successes of the information age through "networked intelligence." The still-young Graphical Internet had demonstrated the power of creating systems with clear rules for contribution – what David Weinberger called "Small pieces loosely joined." This approach enabled millions to experiment and innovate rapidly.

Linux exemplified this phenomenon. Rather than pursuing traditional government contracts and assembling contractors to build an operating system, Linus Torvalds designed the kernel and created clear pathways for contribution. The open-source system quickly became the leading server operating system, spawning profitable companies such as Red Hat Software, valued at $14 billion.

Another inspirational example came from Dee Hock's creation of Visa International. Before the Internet era, Hock conceived a networked organization that became the world's largest commercial financial system. He achieved this by embracing what he called "Chaordia" – a balanced system between rigid control and chaos. Visa didn't issue cards or credit but provided a framework for others to do so under a unified brand, processing billions of transactions valued at over $5 trillion annually.

Three key works shaped my thinking about software architecture: Stephen Wolfram's "A New Kind of Science" taught that simple, clear principles can generate complex, intelligent behavior, while complex rules often yield simple, ineffective outcomes. Nicholas Taleb's "Black Swan" emphasized building resilience into systems that outgrow our ability to track and manage them. Robert Frenay's "Pulse" highlighted nature's mastery of resilient design, showing how biological principles could inform technological systems.

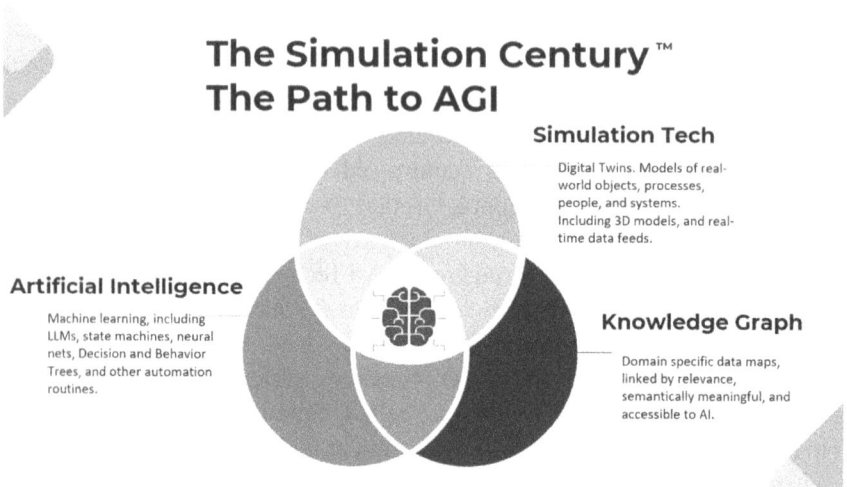

The Simulation Century™
The Path to AGI

Simulation Tech

Digital Twins. Models of real-world objects, processes, people, and systems. Including 3D models, and real-time data feeds.

Artificial Intelligence

Machine learning, including LLMs, state machines, neural nets, Decision and Behavior Trees, and other automation routines.

Knowledge Graph

Domain specific data maps, linked by relevance, semantically meaningful, and accessible to AI.

Figure 1.   The Simulation Century.

This synthesis of ideas suggests a new approach to building complex systems in the accelerating information age – one that embraces networked intelligence, clear principles for contribution, and resilient design inspired by natural systems. As we enter what I call the Simulation Century (see Figure 1), these concepts become increasingly crucial for harnessing artificial intelligence (AI) and simulation technologies to design a better future.

2. The Simulation Century

The 20th century was the first in which humanity could reflect upon past or current events by reviewing video footage. The 20th-century Canadian philosopher Marshall McLuhan developed a theory of media in which he said "the medium is the message." He also said the media we use, in turn, make us. For McLuhan, it was the medium itself that shaped and controlled "the scale and form of human association and action."[1]

If the last century was about the moving image, this century is about simulation. It is the first time in human history when we can employ our newly created super tools including AI and machine learning and also the rich 3D graphical simulation of those worlds in the form of digital twins. With AI-empowered digital twins, we can not only model, simulate, and reflect upon past events and current operations, but we can also now model and simulate complex futures. With this time-traveling capability, we can not only attempt to predict the future but also shape and create the futures we want. This is the highest moral purpose of the age of AI in the Simulation Century.

3. The Information Age in Three Acts

The development of the modern Information Age can be understood through three distinct decades, each characterized by unique technological advances, business models, and societal impacts. This examination explores how each act built upon its predecessor, leading to today's sophisticated integration of AI and human cognition.

---

[1] https://web.mit.edu/allanmc/www/mcluhan.mediummessage.pdf.

4. Act One: 1993–2003 – The Age of Disintermediation

4.1. *The birth of the graphical Internet*

The dawn of the modern Internet era began with the release of Mosaic in 1993, marking a pivotal moment in technological history. Created by Marc Andreessen and his colleagues at the University of Illinois, Mosaic provided the first user-friendly interface to the World Wide Web, transforming what had been a text-based system used primarily by academics into a graphical medium accessible to the general public.

This breakthrough led directly to the creation of Netscape Navigator when Andreessen partnered with Jim Clark to form Netscape Communications. Their decision to release the browser free for non-commercial use proved revolutionary, establishing a model that would influence software distribution for decades to come. The company's spectacular IPO in August 1995 not only launched the dot-com boom but also signaled to the business world that the Internet had become a serious commercial platform.

4.2. *The rise of digital commerce*

During this period, several companies emerged that would fundamentally reshape commerce through disintermediation – the removal of traditional intermediaries from transactions. Amazon, founded in 1994 as an online bookstore, recognized that the Internet could eliminate the need for physical retail locations while offering consumers unprecedented selection. Jeff Bezos's vision of an "everything store" seemed ambitious at the time but proved prescient as Amazon expanded beyond books to become a global retail powerhouse.

eBay, launched in 1995, demonstrated another form of disintermediation by creating a direct marketplace connecting buyers and sellers. The platform's innovation lay in its ability to establish trust through user ratings and reviews, effectively replacing traditional market intermediaries with a community-based reputation system.

PayPal, emerging in 1998, addressed a crucial need in this new digital economy: secure online payments. By providing a trusted intermediary for financial transactions, PayPal paradoxically enabled further disintermediation in other sectors by making digital commerce more accessible and secure.

4.3. *Infrastructure development*

The first act was also marked by massive investments in infrastructure. The dot-com boom, despite its eventual bust, funded the installation of fiber optic networks and data centers that would support future internet growth. Companies such as Cisco, Sun Microsystems, and Oracle provided the hardware and software backbone that made large-scale e-commerce possible.

5. Act Two: 2004–2014 – Capturing and Directing Human Attention

5.1. *The social media revolution*

The second act marked a fundamental shift from disintermediation to attention capture. Facebook, launched from a Harvard dorm room in 2004, initially appeared to be just another social networking site following Friendster and MySpace. However, Mark Zuckerberg's platform introduced several key innovations that would prove transformative:

- the News Feed, which turned user activities into a consumable stream of content,
- the Like button, which provided instant feedback and data collection,
- a platform for third-party applications, turning Facebook into a social operating system.

LinkedIn, while less flashy than Facebook, demonstrated how professional networking could be digitized and monetized. The platform's success showed that social media could serve serious business purposes while still capturing and directing user attention.

5.2. *The search for monetization*

Google's development during this period illustrated the evolution of attention monetization. While the company's search engine had emerged during Act One, it was the development of AdWords and AdSense that transformed Google into a profit machine. These systems perfectly matched the Internet's ability to track user behavior with advertisers' desire for targeted marketing.

Twitter (now X) introduced a new paradigm of real-time, public conversation, though its struggle to find a sustainable business model highlighted the challenges of monetizing attention. The platform's influence on public discourse often exceeded its financial success, demonstrating that attention and monetization don't always align perfectly.

5.3. *Mobile revolution and app economy*

The launch of the iPhone in 2007 and the subsequent smartphone revolution dramatically increased the opportunities for capturing human attention. Mobile devices created new contexts for engagement, leading to services such as Instagram (acquired by Facebook) and Snapchat, which were designed specifically for mobile-first experiences.

6. Act Three: 2015–2022 – Cognitive Coupling and the Noösphere

6.1. *The rise of machine learning*

The third act marked a qualitative shift in human–computer interaction. Advances in machine learning, particularly deep learning and neural networks, enabled new forms of ambient computing. Key developments included the following:

- Natural Language Processing breakthroughs enabling more natural human–computer interaction,
- computer vision advances supporting autonomous vehicles and facial recognition,
- recommendation systems becoming sophisticated enough to predict user preferences accurately.

6.2. *AI assistants and ambient computing*

This period saw the emergence of AI assistants as a new interface paradigm:

- Apple's Siri pioneered voice interaction on mobile devices.
- Amazon's Alexa brought ambient computing into homes.

- Google Assistant demonstrated sophisticated natural language understanding.
- Microsoft's Cortana showed how AI could integrate with productivity tools.

These systems represented the first widespread deployment of AI technologies that could engage in natural conversation with users, marking a significant step toward cognitive coupling between humans and machines.

6.3. The dawn of the Noösphere

The concept of the Noösphere, first proposed by Vladimir Vernadsky and Teilhard de Chardin, describes a sphere of human thought and knowledge enveloping the earth, similar to the atmosphere or biosphere. The third act of the Information Age began to make this concept tangible through the following:

- ubiquitous internet connectivity,
- cloud computing and storage,
- edge computing and IoT devices,
- advanced machine learning systems.

These developments created a genuine global network of human and machine intelligence, leading to what some researchers call "intelligence amplification" – the enhancement of human cognitive capabilities through technological means.

6.4. Implications for the future

As we move beyond Act Three into what might be called the Simulation Century, several key developments are emerging:

1. the integration of AI into every aspect of human activity,
2. the development of sophisticated digital twins for physical systems,
3. the emergence of new interfaces between human and machine intelligence,
4. the potential for predictive modeling of complex systems.

These advancements suggest that the next phase will focus not just on cognitive coupling but also on the active co-evolution of human and machine intelligence. This raises both opportunities and challenges:

* the need for ethical frameworks governing AI development,
* questions about privacy and data ownership,
* the importance of maintaining human agency in automated systems,
* the potential for unprecedented problem-solving capabilities.

The three acts of the Information Age have laid the groundwork for a new era of human–machine collaboration. Understanding this history is crucial for anyone seeking to shape the future of technology and society.

The period after November 30, 2022, is the true dawn of the Simulation Century.

7. Knowledge Graphs: The Memex Cornerstone of Our AI Future

Perhaps the most overlooked element of our new infatuation with large language models trained on the open Internet is the knowledge on which it was trained. LLMs famously are black boxes. They have no software debugger (as of this date) and are not transparent to inquiry. For government organizations, companies, and even individuals, it is important to understand what Sam Adams of IBM coined the 4Vs of the data being mined. The Volume, Variety, Veracity, and even the Velocity of that information are critical to making decisions on how much one should depend on the output of any intelligence derived from that data. For reasons of utility and control and a host of other reasons, it is important to develop and maintain knowledge graphs that are bound by your organization's context (because semantic mistakes still occur and may lead to ML hallucination) and are expertly curated for the purpose they will serve.

We are in an accelerating Information Age. We are creating more information every day than we have available storage. What are we losing every day? Was it important? Was it redundant and trivial and of no consequence that it was lost? The answer to these and so many more Information Age questions lies in the context. In the Information Age after the dawn of machine learning, having a knowledge graph specific to the context of your business or domain is critical.

In his 1945 article in the Atlantic Monthly titled "As We May Think,"[2] Vannevar Bush laid the cornerstone for much of our methods of storage and retrieval and organizations of information. This article was the seed of hypertext links and led to work on ontologies and ultimately to methods for graphing humanity's knowledge.

So, what is a knowledge graph, and how does one go about creating one? Google is credited with popularizing the term knowledge graph beginning in 2012. The Google knowledge graph comprises over 500 million information objects, each graphed in multidimensional space to help its algorithms discern the semantic differences between information objects that have similar names but different contexts. The example IBM gives on its website is of apple the fruit and Apple the computer company. These information object concepts share the same word and even have similar imagery associated with them across the networked intelligence of the Internet but have divergent meanings. In a knowledge graph, these two information objects would be dimensionally far apart in topic node space.

Knowledge graphs are traditionally composed of nodes, edges, and labels. Nodes are the main concepts, edges represent relationships, and labels are the weighted tags on each information object. One of the first projects where this author worked on a knowledge graph was for the Department of Education. In 2010, the Secretary of Education, Arne Duncan, began a project to digitally transform all of the knowledge in the Library of Congress, the Smithsonian, and other government repositories of information. The project was called The Learning Registry.[3,4] Its lofty goal was to make all of the knowledge and objects stored in these catacombs transparent to inquiry across the US education system. Naturally, the first step was scanning all of the books, documents, and artifacts across those collections. As intimidating and laborious as that process was, it paled in comparison to the Sisyphean task of semantically tagging all of those information objects so that they could be matched with those searching for information.

Initially, as items were scanned, experts were asked to tag these items with descriptive hashtags so that they could be categorized. It soon

---

[2] https://www.w3.org/History/1945/vbush/vbush0.shtml.

[3] Advanced Distributed Learning (ADL) Initiative. (n.d.). Learning Registry. ADL Initiative, U.S. Department of Defense. Retrieved May 9, 2025, from https://www.adlnet.gov/projects/learning-registry/, MLA 9th Edition.

[4] https://adlnet.gov/projects/learning-registry/.

became evident that the pace of expert tagging was going to be enormous. Lockheed Martin was asked to flex its new machine learning skills by designing a system that could learn from everything previously tagged and auto tag documents and objects, along with a confidence score based on the amount of training data on each item. If the confidence score was below a certain threshold, the system would notify experts to reinforce its learning by agreeing or editing the tags. Very soon the system grew in its confidence and could auto tag most of the items it encountered. But it really became interesting when it expanded its tagging.

Ontologies: At the time, ontologies were all the rage. In order to aid any expert system, it was standard practice to use a knowledge graph with an ontology specific to the domain area to help the machines in their discernment. Systems such as the W3C's OWL[5] or Web Ontology Language were the standard for representing knowledge in either a vector or graph database. It is important to understand that an ontology is more than just a mapping; it includes logic that describes the meaning of information objects. The graph or vector database is a place to structurally store those representations. Many today think that LLMs have obviated the need for ontologies, but they should be strongly considered in any system that has a specific and critical use case.

The breakthrough during the Learning Registry project was the dramatic difference in scale in having a machine learning system tag information rather than humans. The advantage that machines have is their incredible computation ability. The dramatic improvements in Moore's law over the last decade meant that we had easy access to vast amounts of compute power as well as storage. While a human expert might read Tolstoy's *War and Peace* and tag it with #Russiannovel #Tolstoy #LoveStory #War and perhaps a few other items such as time period and other genre tags, machine systems such as the one for the Learning Registry initially tagged everything with up to 999 weighted tags. In other words, it used the Dewey Decimal System as its ontology and also applied a weight to each topic it assigned. In later projects, we came to call this a "hyperdimensional fingerprint." To humans, this tagging and weighting seems like overkill, but to machines, it is trivial and proved extraordinarily helpful in training the next stage of machine learning systems, particularly natural language processing systems such as LLMs.

---

[5]https://www.w3.org/OWL/.

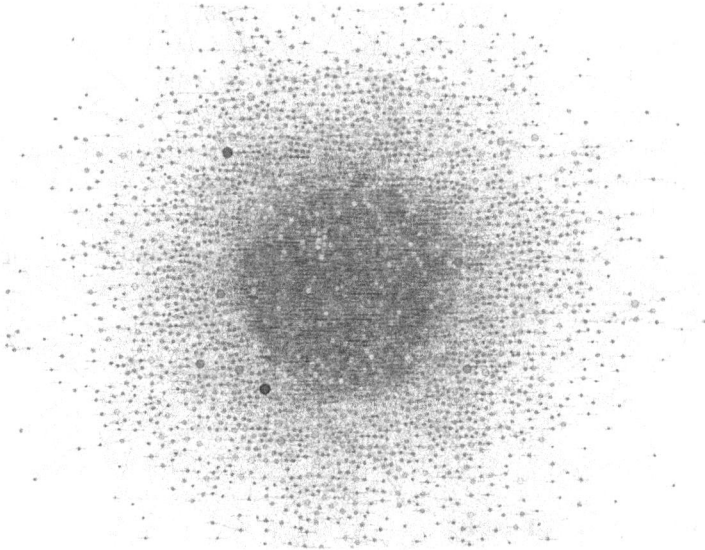

Figure 2. Covid Brain Knowledge Graph built by Tanjo Inc. for a major health insurance company at the beginning of the pandemic.

It is important to understand that, as powerful as machine learning systems and LLMs are proving themselves to be, they can still use help from us in order to perform the utility functions we are asking them to perform. If a company has a good solid ontological mapping of its organizational information and can overlay that on its own knowledge graph in context (see Figure 2), extraordinary capabilities emerge when chatbots are connected to permit companies to "talk to their data."

8. The New Scientific Method

Although AI is like other technologies in many respects, it is unusual in a few important dimensions. Specifically, AI is both a general purpose technology (GPT) – i.e., it has a wide domain of applications – as well as an "invention of a method of invention" (IMI) (Cockburn *et al.*, 2018; Agrawal *et al.*, 2018). Cockburn *et al.* asserted that "… the arrival of a general purpose IMI is a sufficiently uncommon occurrence that its impact could be profound for economic growth and its broader impact on society." They assemble and analyze the corpus of scientific papers and patenting activity in AI and provide evidence consistent with the characterization of machine learning as both a GPT and an IMI.

One such superpower that emerges from machine intelligence with access to big data and knowledge graphs is what we call the new scientific method. The old scientific method, by way of comparison, involves a human expert (presumably a scientist) who dreams up one or more hypotheses they would like to explore. Once they settle on a hypothesis, they would design one or more experiments, run those experiments, observe their results, produce synthesis, and refine their thesis.

With our new machine learning powers, we can provide our systems with large amounts of data and guide them by simply asking them to find "every hypothesis that may be useful". This step sounds trite but is extraordinary in that we are now asking the machine for its perspective.

9. The Big Data Leap

In 2009, Alex Kipman at Microsoft Research Labs in San Francisco was building a dramatically new way for humans to interface with machines. The secret project was called Natal,[6] named for the Brazilian region from which he hailed. The system came to be known as the Microsoft Kinect and consisted of a separate piece of hardware that would interface with the Microsoft xBoxes already shipped all over the world. The system used a very advanced sensor array to detect and map the movements of game players and allow their bodies to become the input device for games. The project faced numerous computer science and hardware challenges. One of the most challenging was that the " brain of the system would have to reside within about 100 MB of available memory on the millions of already shipped xBoxes. The sensor array problem was solved by using the array from the Israeli company Prime Sense. But the final leap was a perplexing computation problem.

In 2009, we still had difficulty with sensors on vehicles to achieve even the lowest level of autonomous driving. The living room and identifying different human problems for the Kinect was a similar issue. At this very early time for AI, researchers were still attempting to solve problems using the "old AI." The old AI meant that the human coder or

---

[6] https://www.wired.com/story/the-game-changer/.

researcher had to thoroughly understand the problem, then code the rigid logic into a finite state machine or behavior tree or set of logic and decision IF, Then/Else code to tell the machine what to do. The reason the DARPA Grand Challenge for autonomous vehicles in 2004 failed so miserably is that researchers had great difficulty in rendering into code how humans drive cars. If we can't articulate how humans make complex decisions in real time while driving, we have no hope of telling a machine how to do it in old AI code. Furthermore, we have since realized that machines don't drive cars the way humans do. Machines have different inputs and outputs. They have LIDAR, GPS, optical sensors, and other methods to detect environmental change and adjust the controls for the vehicle. In 2009, the process of helping a machine recognize the differences between different humans and the cluttered items that might be present in different living rooms around the world in differing lighting conditions was computationally just as out of bounds as the DARPA autonomous vehicle challenge. Alex solved it with machine learning.

Alex had invited Lockheed Martin Virtual World Labs to his lab in 2009 during the Game Developers Conference. This author, who happened to be the Director of LM VWL at the time, arrived prepared to help with the sensors using our Lockheed deep bench on sensor arrays and systems engineering. We quickly realized the Prime Sense structured light system was going to do the trick but stuck around to learn more about this machine learning approach his team was employing. Instead of writing logic code and creating lookup tables, the Kinect team (see Figure 3) was feeding imagery from all over the world into an ML training system. Millions of example images and videos were used. The training back then was very CPU intensive as we did not yet have ML libraries that could take full advantage of the massively parallel processing in GPUs. The process required over 224,000 hours of CPU compute time to create the ML "brain" of the system. The resulting brain fit in less than 60 MB of memory.

Another remarkable piece of this project that fits into our next discussion is that this was not a natural language processing LLM system. It would soon be installed in living rooms all over the world and would be able to sense, see, and hear everything that was happening in those rooms while people used it to play games. And it was processing those inputs.

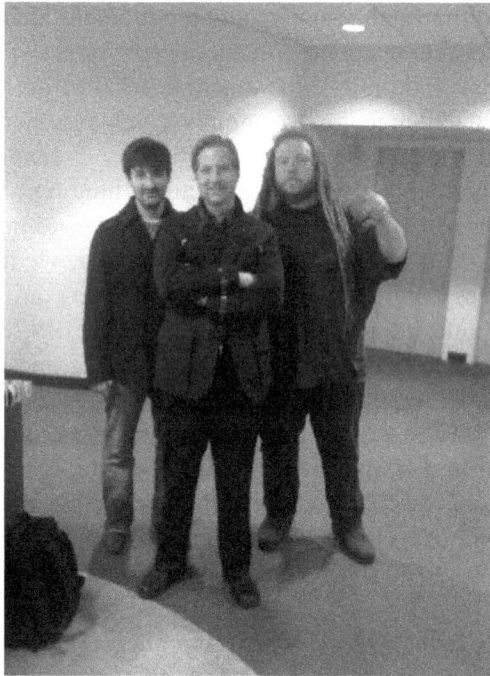

Figure 3. The author Richard Boyd with Microsoft Kinect inventor Alex Kipman and VR pioneer Jaron Lanier. Microsoft Research Labs, San Francisco, 2009.

10. Feeding Your Knowledge Graph: The Narrow Waist for AI Data

10.1. *Data is the critical resource for AI*

AI has the promise to make business operations far more efficient, uncovering hidden cost savings, showing when and where products and services will be demanded, and finding hidden gems among people and operations.

It does this by analyzing data from a company's operations and sales and fusing it with data from external sources – freely available public datasets and published data from customers, suppliers, and competitors. Analysis of all of that data can show surprising correlations and trends, everything from periodicities in equipment efficiency to supply crunches due to weather events to the sensitivity of demand to interest rates and currency fluctuations and much more. In fact, AI, at the end of the day, is extremely intensive processing of vast quantities of data, and it is the exponential growth in data that genuinely powers the AI revolution. Dr. Peter Norvig, head of Google Research and the co-author of the leading textbook on AI, noted that Google's AI techniques aren't better than everyone else's – but Google's unmatched ability to gather and process vast amounts of data gives it the edge. Data is the key to AI, which is why it's said that data is the new oil.

AI experts around the world point to the criticality of data for AI. Shub Bhowmick, CEO of Tredence, says that in order to see the value of AI "stakeholders must ensure a solid data foundation that enables the full cycle of data management, embrace advanced analytical methods to realize the untapped value of data." Moses Guttman, CEO of ClearML, says, "AI requires meaningful data to make noticeable improvements and drive commercial innovation." Umesh Sachdev, CEO of Uniphore, notes that the critical factor in AI success is "availability and access to data; and understanding how to apply that data to specific use cases to improve business outcomes."

But despite its promise, data is hard to get. This is the AI paradox – AI is a well-tuned machine designed to process data, but finding the data to fuel the AI machine is not easy. So, data is the new oil in two ways – like oil, it fuels the engine of growth. And like oil, it must be found, mined, and refined. Your company or organization is AI ready when it has a process for finding, mining, and refining the data needed to generate insights about your business and the environment in which it operates.

Why is this? Because data is almost always generated as a byproduct of other operations, and these operations rarely consider the value of the data that they produce. Consider, for example, a registration system at a hotel. The system is designed to register guests, get them to an appropriate available room, and collect payment information. It's not designed to generate demographic information on who is renting rooms of which type on which seasons or days. That information is enormously valuable – but the system doesn't collect it or make it available easily.

This is replicated hundreds of times throughout your business. Text fields in inventory databases describe items in (often brief) form, but this isn't readily available for processing. "I have Diet Coke under multiple SKUs in my database, but I don't even know which ones," the Chief Information Officer of Safeway complained. "All of the information I need to design personalized instructional curricula for my students is in our registration system, but it's impossible to get at," said the Chief Data Officer of a major university in a private conversation. Much of the information your enterprise needs is locked up in documents on employees' desktop computers; in one business we worked with, sales projections were entered by hand into spreadsheets by each salesperson, and the reps then mailed the spreadsheets to the sales lead's admin for presentation. Tax and expense data is in accounting systems such as QuickBooks, which can generate reports for human consumption, but which really aren't designed for automated processing.

> "AI data readiness is the discovery, mining, and refinement of data into fuel for the AI engine. Organizational AI readiness hinges on policy and change management."

Let us return to the oil analogy. Data *discovery* is the process of finding the data that your enterprise relies on for its operations, and the repositories, applications, and external data sources where it may be found. Data *mining* is the extraction of that data from those sources. Data *refining* is the process of adding information to the data to ready it for AI, typically *metadata* which indicates what the data means.

The AI Data Plane offers a framework for the discovery, mining, refinement, and enhancement of AI data. The AI Readiness Pyramid offers a framework for guiding your enterprise on the path to filling the Data Plane with usable AI.

10.2. *The AI Data Plane*

The AI Data Plane is a framework for *specifying, capturing, and representing* enterprise data. It is the basis of the *AI Data Pipeline* and manages and governs the phases of *discovery, mining, refining,* and *enhancing* enterprise AI data. It treats all data sources uniformly, and, importantly, makes no distinction between an original data source and any of the applications and tools in the data pipeline. In the AI Data Plane Framework, each tool in the AI Data Pipeline simply reads objects from the AI Data Plane and writes a new object into the Data Plane. As a result, each tool or application sees a uniform environment. This is crucial because it permits the rigorous specification of data objects and offers the ability to thoroughly check the functionality and correctness of each tool in the data pipeline. It offers the ability to specify which data and information is critical to an enterprise, and it offers a clean separation of, and independent development of, extraction of data from sources and usage of data in applications. It does this through the **Data Equivalence Principle**: *it is not* *possible, **even in principle**, to determine the source of data from the data itself, or from the applications that use the data.*

The Data Equivalence Principle does for the data pipeline what abstract interfaces and APIs did for application development. Just as abstract interfaces and APIs cleanly separate the function of a software component from its implementation, the Data Equivalence Principle cleanly separates the semantics of the information from its storage or computation.

10.3. *The Data Pipeline*

The *Data Pipeline* is the name for the sequence of transformations that data from multiple sources undergo in order to become the final data product suitable for AI procedures. Before the introduction of the Data Plane and the Data Equivalence Principle, the Data Pipeline was an informal set of connectors and programs; with the introduction of the Data Plane and the Data Equivalence Principle, it is a set of rigorous, testable specifications for each transformation.

10.4. *The Data Interface*

The key element in the data pipeline is the *Data Interface*. This does for data what an Application Programming Interface (API) specification does for a computational service. It specifies the semantics of the data that this data source produces, *without* specifying how the data is produced or stored. This is the exact analog of an API specification, which specifies the API calls to which the service responds, and the form of the responses, *without* specifying the implementation.

In the case of the Data Interface, the specification is of a table – a series (potentially infinite) of fixed-length records. The table is defined by a list of *columns*; each column is a triple: a *name*, a *type* (which must be a string, number, Boolean, date, timestamp, or datetime), and (optionally) a metadata record, which gives the meaning of the column. The Data Interface specification is silent on the fields and values of the metadata record; this is something which must be mutually intelligible to the data receiver and source. Examples of common fields in the metadata record are "units" (for numeric specifications), "null" (a value which should always be read as null for a column), and so on.

10.5. *The Data Twin*

The Data Twin is optional (but highly recommended). It is a simulated Data Source that implements the Data Interface and responds to the standard Data Source API. A Data Twin performs multiple roles in the Data Plane ecosystem:

- Full definition of the semantics of the data represented by the Data Interface. The Data Interface captures the structure of the data; the fields, types of each field, and the semantics expressible as state-free logical constructs (e.g., max, min, allowable values, and units). However, semantics which are state-dependent require a full simulation implementation.
- To permit the development of applications of the Data Interface while the Data Source is being developed. *Because of the Data Equivalence Principle, the Data Twin is indistinguishable from the live Data Source.* As a result, data applications can be developed using the Data Twin and the actual source substituted seamlessly.
- The Data Twin captures the *expected* behavior of the Data Source, which can be used as a test for the behavior of the physical Data Source when the latter is implemented. When the two diverge, either the data is not what's expected or there's a bug in the actual Data Source (the Data Twin is typically so simple that it's error-free). In either case, there's valuable information.
- Using the Data Twin as a sample input environment for data applications exposes any shortcomings in the data interfaces chosen for the data application (e.g., the AI/ML application). *Every computational interface, either functional or data, requires iteration; getting interfaces exactly right the first time is equivalent to hitting the center of a dartboard at 50 meters, blindfolded.* For this reason, computation is an experimental discipline. Data Twins afford the opportunity for rapid, inexpensive experimentation.
- The Data Twin fully expresses the expected semantics of the Data Source and thus can act as a source of tests for the actual Data Source implementation. This is particularly valuable when the actual Data Source is realized as a set of proxies.

The last point is particularly important. One important class of data source is logfiles from applications and websites. In one case for a major online delivery service, an application engineer changed the capitalization of variables reported in a logfile. Business metrics were captured from a series of transformations from the logfiles, and these appeared to suddenly and unexpectedly diverge, causing a significant investigation into the business. After a week, the error was discovered. Had the online delivery service implemented a Data Twin for each data source, the root cause would have been rapidly detected because the specific data source divergence would have been apparent.

10.6. The Data Source

The Data Interface and the Data Twin specify the semantics of the data that a Data Source will serve. The Data Source is the implementation that delivers it. Every Data Source implements the Data Plane API, which is given in high-level form here:

- Return the data's rows that match a filter value, as specified in the Data Plane Filter Language. If only certain columns are specified, only those columns are returned.
- Return the data's column headers, including name, type, and metadata.
- Return the minimum and maximum values for a specific column.
- Return all the distinct values in a column.

The Data Plane is designed to be as simple as possible to implement either a Data Plane sender/server or client/receiver (reference implementations are open-source under a BSD license).
In particular:

- All returns are in JavaScript Object Notation (JSON) format.
- All returns of rows are of the same lengths; there are no distinguished null values since this would complicate the receiver's job.
- The transfer protocol is layered on top of http/https.
- Authentication is done through bearer tokens.

10.7. Using the AI Data Plane

The AI Data Plane is the basis for an enterprise's AI Data Strategy; all data is formalized through a set of Data Interfaces, which are then realized as Data Plane data sources. A Data Plane Data Source can be as simple as a database connector or a set of spreadsheets, with a Data Plane server acting as a front end/server to hide the implementation. Or the Data Plane Data Source can be as complex as a supercomputer running a climate simulation, or anything in between. Per the Data Equivalence Principle, there's no way to tell – the only signature of a Data Plane Data Source is its corresponding Data Interface, *and the Data Interface is completely independent of the Data Source's implementation.*

This leads to a disciplined methodology in constructing an enterprise's Data Plane.

10.8. *Specify the Data Interfaces*

The first step is always defining the data required for the AI application. This involves specifying the Data Interfaces for the AI application. *It is critical that the Data Interfaces for the AI application be defined without regard for the data actually available today.* As we see in the following, there are potentially a number of ways to construct a Data Source for a Data Interface. However, if the Data Interface is limited by the data readily available, the AI applications will be hampered immediately by insufficient data.

When data required for an application is unavailable, proxies of one sort or another are always used. This goes on today. The only question is whether the proxying will be done *explicitly*, in a recognized Data Source, or *implicitly*, as part of the AI application. The latter is what's done today; the former is preferable because it explicitly shows where data is missing and how the missing data is being mitigated and because it permits the introduction of more robust and accurate proxies or means of collecting the ground truth data.

10.9. *Implement Data Twins*

Once the Data Interfaces are defined, the recommended next step is to implement a Data Twin for each Data Interface. As mentioned above, this completes the semantics of the Data Interface.

10.10. *Use AI on Data Twins as a predictor*

At this point, the data application (typically an AI application) can be developed using Data Twin as a substitute for the data source. As mentioned above, it's important to do this before or concurrently with implementing the Data Source because the Data Interface and the Data Twin jointly act as a specification for the Data Source. The Data Source is typically much more complex to implement than the Data Twin because the Data Source has to mine the actual data; so, ensuring that the Data Source is plumbing exactly the right data is vital.

10.11. *Identify and implement Data Sources*

Once the Data Twin has been developed and the application is running well with the Twin, it's time to construct the Data Source. This involves writing the connectors for the various actual data repositories, and at this point, the Data Twin as a validator for the Data Source becomes important.

10.12. *Use AI on implemented Data Sources*

- The AI Application is running smoothly using the Data Twin as its Data Source.
- The Data Source on live data has been implemented.
- The equivalence of the Data Twin and Data Source has been validated.

This is where the power of the Data Equivalence Principle and Data Twins becomes evident. *The AI Application cannot, **even in principle**, determine whether its data is coming from the Twin or the live Source.* So, the final step is almost an anticlimax:

There are flourishes, of course: one can run the Data application over the Data Source and the Data Application over the Data Twin side-by-side to ensure that the performance is equivalent.

10.13. *AI Data readiness levels*

- **Level 0:** Enterprise data in documents, spreadsheets, ERP applications, isolated databases, metadata capture non-existent.
- **Level 1:** Enterprise information expressed as AI Data Plane tables:
  - Metadata for Enterprise AI plane tables complete.
- **Level 2:** AI Data Plane Data Twins constructed for Enterprise AI Data Plane Tables:

    ○ Machine Learning/AI/Enterprise simulations over AI Data Plane Data Twins.
- **Level 3:** Connectors for Enterprise Data Sources to AI Data Plane Tables defined:
  - ○ Rigorous tests for AI Data Plane tables defined and executing.
- **Level 4:** Connectors for Enterprise Data Sources to AI Data Plane Tables implemented:
  - ○ Rigorous Data Plane Data Ops tests executing.
- **Level 5:** AI/ML Procedures running on live Enterprise Data:
  - ○ Rigorous test matches against AI Data Plane Data Twins running.

11. 3D Digital Data Twins and the Simulation Equivalence Principle

One of the most powerful uses of AI and simulation technologies in the Simulation Century is the ability to create Digital Twins of complex systems. As with so many of our technological innovations, there are a variety of implementation options and multiple definitions of digital twins. The highest value case is a Digital Twin that is a data-fed simulation of a complex system or business operation that is bit identical to all of the data emanating from or feeding that system that may also have a three-dimensional graphical simulation twin of that system. In the case of a manufacturing plant, a hospital, or an entire city, there are complexities that are best observed in as many dimensions as possible. X, Y, and Z spatial representations of all of the interworking systems with the added dimension of operation over time create powerful new capabilities. The ability to go back in time to forensically review any event helps gain a better understanding of that event. The ability to review operations in real time provides an operational view that can enhance insights and control. Remote monitoring is especially helpful for areas where it is difficult to achieve comprehensive understanding of an operation where human and camera views are obscured. A digital twin of a Boeing 787 or a 688 attack submarine can allow a human operator to see through virtual walls to track wiring and hydraulic systems and zoom in and out to track processes. But the most powerful capability is the potential to travel into the future to not only predict or rehearse future events but also use the AI-powered Digital Twin to design the most desirable future outcomes.

12. The Six Levels of AI Application and the Highest Moral Purpose

Since November 30, 2022, we have been experiencing a seismic shift around the globe. The practice of feeding large amounts of digital data into machine learning neural nets and large language models is creating new opportunities not just for the automation of human cognitive and physical work but also for unlocking new methods for humanity to reflect on the natural and manmade world. And now that the Simulation Century has fully dawned, we have the potential to enlist these new powers in the service of designing better systems, better cities, and better-governing structures.

Leveraging decades of experience working with AI, I've identified six progressive stages that act as a road map from simple automation to genuinely transformative impacts of this evolving technology. We'll begin this journey in our current phase, the "Chat Era," and work our way forward, learning the challenges and possibilities in designing our future for the greatest good.

12.1. *Stage 1: Chat – The dawn of conversational companions*

We find ourselves at an exciting inflection point in the evolution of AI. In the Chat Era, AI has shed its old skin of basic, scripted responses to emerge as a versatile conversationalist capable of much more than a simple Q&A session. Chatbots have transformed our interaction with the digital world, humanizing the technology we've used for years. By harnessing the full potential of AI chat systems built upon large language models, we can enhance production and create efficiencies across every area of human endeavor. Chatbots can provide real-time updates on production statuses and delivery dates manufacturing, reducing operational costs and improving customer satisfaction, contributing to an agile and responsive supply chain. To transition gracefully into the next stage of AI – content creation – AI must deepen its understanding of complex human interactions. It's about evolving past basic keyword recognition to grasp the nuances of language and context. Most importantly, upholding stringent ethical standards in data collection and use is imperative, ensuring user trust and privacy are always maintained.

12.2. *Stage 2: Content creation – The double-edged sword*

With the second stage of AI development, AI's capabilities in content creation spark tremendous excitement and ethical concerns. AI's proficiency in tasks such as drafting legal documents and performing homework assignments for students and written correspondence or creating digital artwork marks a giant leap in productivity and creativity. However, as AI begins to shoulder more cognitive responsibilities, it's become clear this advancement is not without dilemma. In particular, the convenience of relying on AI for creative and analytical tasks could inadvertently weaken our critical-thinking skills, relegating us to the role of technology supervisors rather than active creators. We must learn to prompt AI for productivity without relying on it for all original creation. Then, there's the moral landscape of AI-generated content. Now that we have technologies capable of producing hyper realistic fake images and audio, the potential for misuse skyrockets. Scammers can now create convincing forgeries that can be used to spread misinformation or commit fraud, posing serious challenges to ethical norms and legal frameworks. We must develop robust systems to monitor and evaluate AI outputs to advance our collective goals, not hinder them.

12.3. *Stage 3: Work efficiency – The automation advantage*

Process and workflow automation isn't a new concept, but recent advances have elevated it to new levels of efficiency and intelligence. While traditional automation handles straightforward tasks, modern systems redefine processes, manage complex workflows, and analyze vast volumes of data with remarkable speed and accuracy. Beyond administrative efficiency, these advancements are transforming the workplace by reallocating routine and repetitive tasks to machines, freeing up humans for higher-order thinking and creative problem-solving. This shift can boost productivity while enhancing job satisfaction so workers can focus on more engaging and meaningful work. The key to these transitions is thoughtful integration, ensuring automation complements rather than replaces human expertise.

12.4. *Stage 4: Prediction – Navigating the Simulation Century™*

A huge leap for humanity in the Simulation Century™ is the ability to deeply model complex systems and predict outcomes far in advance. Understanding not only the first-order consequences but also the second, third, fourth, and beyond consequences of an action is a superhuman power. Digital twins and knowledge graphs have become essential tools, offering detailed simulations of physical processes and systemic interactions. Digital twins, for instance, allow cities to test and refine systems virtually before implementation, greatly enhancing urban efficiency and safety. Similarly, in the manufacturing industry, they can predict equipment failures before they occur, minimizing downtime and extending machinery life. Knowledge graphs complement these simulations by mapping intricate organizational data into relevant and actionable insights, aiding in swift, strategic decision-making. This stage of the AI journey requires a sophisticated blend of human and machine intelligence in which predictive capabilities surpass reactivity and enable organizations to analyze potential outcomes with remarkable precision.

12.5. Stage 5: Improved judgment – Harnessing AI for better decisions

Improved judgment is the ultimate goal of AI and machine learning technology. Daniel Kahneman said a decade ago that in the machine age, every organization should allocate 1% of its budget to modeling its actions and improving judgment. This critical capability is being overlooked in the ChatGPT era of talking to data and effortlessly producing content, much of which could be prone to hallucination or of questionable value when not paired with a contextually bound and curated knowledge graph. AI's potential to supplement human judgment, particularly through tools such as knowledge graphs, is an untapped treasure in decision-making processes. Influential thinkers such as Kahneman emphasize AI's significant value in areas requiring complex decision-making, such as governance and public policy. Knowledge graphs visually organize extensive datasets, helping decision-makers find connections and patterns that inform better judgments. Integrating AI with human intuition creates a powerful synergy, making decisions more comprehensive and forward-thinking.

12.6. Stage 6: Designing the future – AI as a force for good

The final stage of AI development is about harnessing AI to shape outcomes that benefit society deliberately. As I've often emphasized, the ultimate moral purpose of technology is not merely to predict complex future outcomes but to actively design the future we desire. We can create and work toward achieving our aspirational goals by harnessing AI. Alan Kay once said, "The best way to predict the future is to invent it." In this spirit, we use AI not just as a tool for forecasting but as a fundamental force in shaping a future aligned with our highest ethical standards. On this front, the adoption of AI paired with digital twin simulations of the real world offers substantial possibilities. AI's ability to advance sustainable and efficient production can be transformative. This vision of AI as a catalyst for good emphasizes the importance of proactive design. It challenges us to think creatively and responsibly about how we program and deploy AI, ensuring it positively contributes to our collective future. Through such efforts, AI can help us navigate and shape the complexities of the modern world, making it a better place for future generations.

12.7. *Envisioning tomorrow: The expansive future of AI*

As we journey through the Simulation Century™ and its possibilities, we should focus on technological advancement and how these technologies can be harnessed to reflect our highest societal and ethical values. AI offers more than efficiency and convenience; it presents an opportunity to design a future that embraces sustainability, equity, and human dignity. The path we pave with AI today will dictate the landscape of tomorrow, challenging us to envision and strive for a future that transcends our current limitations.

References

Digital twin technology and simulation: benefits, usage and predictions 2018. *I-Scoop* (accessed November 11, 2017).

Elisa, N. (2017). A review of the roles of Digital Twin in CPS-based production systems. *Procedia Manufacturing*, *11*, 939–948.

Gelernter, D. H. (1991). *Mirror Worlds: or the Day Software Puts the Universe in a Shoebox – How It Will Happen and What It Will Mean*. Oxford University Press, New York.

Grieves, M. (2015). Can the digital twin transform manufacturing, October 5. World Economic Forum Emerging Technologies (accessed November 19, 2022).

The Gemini Principles (2018). Centre for Digital Built Britain (accessed January 1, 2020).

https://doi.org/10.1142/9789819813506_0007

Chapter 7

Bridging the Gap: Overcoming Integration and Interoperability Challenges in Digital Healthcare Systems

Alexeis Garcia Perez

Aston University, Birmingham, UK

1. Introduction

The digital transformation of healthcare represents a critical response to the rising demand for efficient, accessible, and personalized medical services (Colther and Doussoulin, 2024). Globally, healthcare systems are transitioning from traditional methods to more technology-driven models, leveraging innovations, such as electronic health records (EHRs), tele-medicine, and wearable health devices. This shift, accelerated by the COVID-19 pandemic, underscores the need for digital tools to ensure continuity of care during crises. However, integrating these technologies into existing healthcare frameworks presents significant challenges (Kaye *et al.*, 2024).

Several recent studies (e.g., Tolley *et al.*, 2023; Costa *et al.*, 2024; Abima *et al.*, 2024; Sun, 2024) identify overcoming barriers to integration and interoperability of disparate healthcare systems as a primary issue. Integration entails combining various subsystems or technologies into a cohesive whole, while interoperability focuses on enabling these subsystems to exchange and utilize information seamlessly. These challenges limit the full potential of digital healthcare systems, often constraining providers' ability to deliver comprehensive and coordinated care.

This chapter addresses these integration and interoperability challenges within digital healthcare systems, exploring technological, organizational, and policy-related barriers that hinder seamless data sharing. Building on the author's work on this domain (e.g., Martinez-Caro *et al.*, 2017; Garcia-Perez *et al.*, 2023), and through a synthesis of a case study and conceptual models, this chapter identifies contributing factors and offers potential solutions. By examining both theoretical perspectives and real-world examples, it aims to provide valuable insights for academics and practitioners striving to overcome these obstacles.

This chapter begins by defining integration and interoperability in the context of digital healthcare systems. It then examines the technological, organizational, and regulatory barriers to progress in this domain. A case study illustrates practical challenges and solutions, followed by a discussion of strategies to enhance integration and interoperability through technological innovations, collaborative efforts, and policy recommendations. Throughout, evidence-based insights and practical guidance are offered to healthcare providers and stakeholders working to optimize the functionality and effectiveness of digital health systems.

2. Defining Integration and Interoperability in Healthcare

2.1. *Conceptualizing integration and interoperability*

Integration and interoperability are cornerstone concepts in the digital transformation of healthcare systems (Engel *et al.*, 2006). Though often used interchangeably, these terms carry distinct meanings and implications.

Integration refers to the process of combining various technologies, systems, and data sources into a unified, seamless ecosystem. In digital healthcare, this involves connecting diverse software applications, databases, and medical devices to function cohesively, enabling healthcare professionals to access and share information across platforms. Integration aims to create a holistic view of patient data, enhancing decision-making, care coordination, and overall patient outcomes (Wessels *et al.*, 2010).

For example, integration might link a hospital's patient management system with laboratory information systems or connect EHRs with telemedicine platforms.

Interoperability, by contrast, concerns the capacity of different systems and devices to communicate and exchange data in a standardized, meaningful manner. Achieving true interoperability requires using common data standards, such as HL7 or FHIR (Fast Healthcare Interoperability Resources), ensuring data can be shared and interpreted consistently across platforms (Benson and Grieve, 2016; Mandel *et al.*, 2016). Without interoperability, technological integration remains fragmented, hampering effective data exchange and collaborative care.

While integration emphasizes the technical unification of systems, interoperability underscores the utility and coherence of shared data. Both dimensions are indispensable for seamless digital healthcare operations and their interplay underpins the transformative potential of digital health solutions.

2.2. *Importance in digital transformation*

Integration and interoperability are pivotal for improving patient care, operational efficiency, and the delivery of personalized treatment. Wearable health monitors, remote consultations, and AI-powered diagnostics exemplify digital solutions that rely on interconnected systems for real-time data sharing. For instance, wearable devices such as specific smart watches may transmit vital health data to providers, while remote consultations leverage integrated EHRs to offer comprehensive patient histories (Abbas *et al.*, 2021; El-Rashidy *et al.*, 2021). Such capabilities are especially critical when patients receive care across various settings (e.g., hospitals and clinics) and home care.

Telemedicine in rural areas illustrates the importance of interoperability. Local clinics may conduct routine checks, but specialists in distant locations require real-time access to patients' medical histories for effective consultation (Moffatt and Eley, 2011). Without interoperable systems, manual data transfers slow processes, increasing the risk of errors and inefficiencies. Conversely, interoperable systems facilitate instantaneous data sharing, enabling informed, timely decisions that improve health outcomes.

Advanced technologies such as AI and machine learning (ML) further highlight the reliance on interoperability. AI algorithms demand comprehensive datasets to deliver accurate insights. When data is scattered across non-interoperable systems, the effectiveness of these algorithms is reduced, limiting their transformative potential (Reddy *et al.*, 2019; Jiang *et al.*, 2017).

2.3. *Frameworks for integration and interoperability*

Guiding frameworks for integration and interoperability often address both technical and organizational facets. HL7's FHIR standard, for instance, simplifies data exchange using web technologies and has gained traction for bridging legacy and modern systems (HL7 International, 2021). OpenEHR, another significant framework, structures data around patient-centric health records accessible to authorized providers (OpenEHR Foundation, 2021; Wollersheim *et al.*, 2009).

Organizational frameworks complement these technical solutions by fostering collaboration among stakeholders, from healthcare providers to technology developers, policymakers, and patients. Cross-sector partnerships align stakeholder needs, ensuring sustainability and scalability (Taylor *et al.*, 2020; Johnson and Smith, 2019).

Achieving integration and interoperability requires addressing complex technical and organizational factors. Success lies in unifying diverse technologies while ensuring effective communication among systems to enable seamless information flow.

3. Barriers to Effective Integration and Interoperability

Despite the clear advantages of integrated and interoperable healthcare systems, significant barriers persist in their implementation. These barriers are multifaceted, encompassing technological, organizational, and regulatory dimensions, each contributing to the fragmentation of healthcare delivery and hindering the realization of seamless digital transformation.

3.1. *Technological barriers*

One of the foremost challenges lies in the technological fragmentation of healthcare systems. Many organizations rely on legacy systems that lack the capacity for modern integration. Over the years, these systems have often operated using proprietary data formats and outdated protocols, rendering them incompatible with newer technologies (Vest and Gamm, 2010; Adere, 2022). The absence of universally adopted standards exacerbates this issue, as systems developed by different vendors fail to communicate effectively.

Interoperability is further hindered by the lack of investment in updated infrastructure. Healthcare organizations frequently operate under tight budget constraints, prioritizing immediate clinical needs over long-term technological upgrades. This underinvestment results in systems that are not only outdated but also incapable of supporting the data-intensive demands of modern healthcare, such as AI-powered analytics and telemedicine platforms.

3.2. *Organizational barriers*

Organizational factors also present substantial challenges. Resistance to change among healthcare professionals is a critical issue, driven by a lack of training and unfamiliarity with new technologies (Taylor *et al.*, 2020). Healthcare staff often perceive digital transformation initiatives as disruptive to established workflows, leading to reluctance to adopt new systems.

Moreover, the siloed nature of many healthcare organizations limits collaborative efforts to achieve integration. Departments often operate independently, utilizing disparate systems that are not designed for inter-connectivity. This fragmentation limits data sharing and undermines the potential for comprehensive patient care.

3.3. *Regulatory barriers*

The regulatory landscape adds another layer of complexity. Stringent data privacy laws, such as the General Data Protection Regulation (GDPR) in the European Union, impose rigorous requirements on data handling (European Commission, 2018). While these regulations are essential for safeguarding patient information, they can also slow the adoption of interoperable systems.

Additionally, the lack of harmonized policies across jurisdictions poses challenges for cross-border interoperability. In an increasingly globalized world, patients often seek healthcare services in multiple countries. However, varying standards and legal frameworks create obstacles to seamless data exchange, limiting the effectiveness of international healthcare networks.

3.4. *Cybersecurity concerns*

Cybersecurity risks further complicate the integration process. As healthcare systems become more interconnected, they also become more vulnerable to cyber threats (Garcia-Perez *et al.*, 2023). Data breaches not only compromise patient privacy but also erode trust in digital health solutions (Rosa *et al.*, 2019). Addressing these risks requires significant investment in robust security measures, which many organizations struggle to afford.

Addressing these barriers demands a comprehensive approach that considers the interplay of technological, organizational, and regulatory factors. The following sections explores strategies and frameworks that can help overcome these challenges, drawing on both theoretical insights and practical examples.

4. Case Study: Overcoming Challenges

To illustrate the real-world challenges and solutions associated with achieving integration and interoperability in healthcare systems, this section presents a case study of a healthcare institution that embarked on a comprehensive digital transformation initiative (Martínez-Caro *et al.*, 2018). The institution in question is a mid-sized hospital network in Spain that undertook an ambitious project to integrate its healthcare services, including primary care, emergency care, laboratory systems, and telemedicine platforms.

4.1. *Case study context*

The hospital network had relied on a mix of legacy IT systems for years, with separate systems for patient management, laboratory results, and medical imaging. These systems were not interoperable, leading to inefficiencies and fragmented care delivery. For example, physicians in the emergency department (ED) faced challenges accessing patients' medical histories, making it difficult to make informed decisions quickly during critical situations. Additionally, patients visiting different specialists across the network often had to repeat tests and provide the same personal health information multiple times, causing frustration and delays.

4.2. Challenges faced

One significant challenge was the integration of disparate legacy systems. Each department used its own IT solutions, many of which were decades old and lacked standardized data formats or protocols. Integrating these systems into a cohesive digital infrastructure required substantial technical effort, as each system operated in isolation and used proprietary formats that hindered communication.

Another barrier was the lack of interoperability between the hospital's telemedicine platform and its EHR system. Although the telemedicine platform enabled remote consultations with specialists, it could not seamlessly exchange patient data with the EHR. This meant that physicians conducting remote consultations were unable to access up-to-date patient records or test results in real time, reducing the effectiveness of telemedicine and delaying diagnosis and treatment.

Cybersecurity concerns further compounded the integration process. As the hospital network explored ways to connect its various systems and expand data sharing, protecting sensitive patient information became a critical priority. The sheer volume of data and variety of systems involved posed significant risks, necessitating robust security measures to prevent breaches and maintain patient trust.

4.3. Approaches and solutions

To overcome these challenges, the hospital network adopted a multipronged strategy that combined technological and organizational solutions:

1. *Adoption of interoperability standards*: The hospital implemented the FHIR standard, an open framework for electronic data exchange that simplifies integration by using modern web technologies, such as RESTful APIs. FHIR allowed previously incompatible systems to exchange data in a consistent format, bridging gaps between the telemedicine platform and the EHR system. This real-time data exchange significantly improved the efficiency and quality of remote consultations.

2. *Implementation of a unified data platform to address data fragmentation*: The hospital introduced a unified data platform that integrated various services, including EHRs, lab systems, and medical imaging. This open-architecture platform centralized patient data, ensuring healthcare professionals could access comprehensive information for clinical decision-making. Advanced analytics capabilities also enabled predictive insights, such as identifying patients at risk of readmission.
3. *Cybersecurity enhancements*: The hospital strengthened its security framework by implementing end-to-end encryption for data transmissions and adopting multifactor authentication protocols. Regular security audits and staff training programs ensured adherence to best practices. Collaborating with cybersecurity experts helped identify vulnerabilities and mitigate risks, bolstering trust among staff and patients.

4.4. Outcomes and lessons learned

The efforts of the hospital network resulted in notable improvements in care delivery and operational efficiency. Physicians gained timely access to patient information, enabling quicker and more accurate diagnoses. Patients experienced reduced redundancy in tests and consultations, enhancing satisfaction with the healthcare system. The implementation of robust security measures further ensured compliance with data protection regulations and safeguarded patient trust.

This case study underscores the importance of adopting interoperability standards, investing in modern infrastructure, and addressing organizational and cybersecurity challenges. The strategies employed by the hospital serve as a model for other healthcare organizations seeking to achieve successful digital transformation.

5. Strategies for Improving Integration and Interoperability

Achieving effective integration and interoperability in healthcare systems is a multifaceted challenge, requiring targeted strategies across technological, organizational, and policy domains. This section explores several key strategies that healthcare organizations can implement to overcome barriers and enhance the seamless integration of digital systems. These strategies are drawn from best practices, case studies, and emerging trends in healthcare technology.

5.1. *Technological solutions*

Technological solutions for improving integration and interoperability focus on standardization, modern infrastructure, and emerging technologies. These approaches enable healthcare organizations to connect disparate systems and ensure that patient data flows seamlessly across different platforms.

The adoption of open standards and interoperability protocols is one of the most critical steps in achieving interoperability. For instance, the FHIR standard provides a flexible and efficient way for healthcare systems to exchange data. By using modern web-based technologies, such as RESTful APIs, FHIR enables communication between systems in a standardized manner. This makes FHIR an invaluable tool for bridging the gap between legacy systems and newer technologies (Mandel *et al.*, 2016). In addition to FHIR, standards such as HL7 (Health Level 7) and IHE (Integrating the Healthcare Enterprise) play pivotal roles in ensuring data exchange. These frameworks reduce the need for custom integrations and improve data usability across the healthcare ecosystem (Benson and Grieve, 2016).

Cloud computing has become a cornerstone of modern healthcare IT infrastructure. By storing data in the cloud, healthcare organizations can facilitate the integration of different systems regardless of location or technical specifications. Centralized cloud platforms allow healthcare providers to access medical records, test results, and other patient information in real time. Cloud-based systems also promote collaboration among healthcare providers. For example, a patient's primary care doctor, specialist, and pharmacist can all access the same cloud-based medical record, improving care coordination and reducing errors. Built-in security features, such as data encryption and multifactor authentication, enhance data protection while enabling easier data sharing (Ehwerhemuepha *et al.*, 2020).

Emerging technologies such as artificial intelligence (AI) and ML are increasingly vital for improving integration and interoperability. AI can process and analyze vast amounts of healthcare data, while ML algorithms help predict health outcomes, identify patterns, and suggest treatment options based on patients' medical histories. AI and ML also enhance interoperability by automating data extraction and processing. For instance, AI-driven algorithms can convert unstructured data such as clinical notes or medical images into structured formats, simplifying data sharing and analysis across multiple sources (Reddy *et al.*, 2019; Jiang *et al.*, 2017).

5.2. Collaborative strategies

Successful integration and interoperability require collaboration among healthcare providers, IT professionals, policymakers, and patients.

Collaboration between healthcare providers and technology developers ensures the creation of solutions that meet stakeholders' needs. IT professionals must work closely with healthcare providers to design user-friendly digital systems, addressing issues related to usability, data quality, and workflow disruptions (Taylor *et al.*, 2020). Public–private partnerships also foster innovation and sustainability. Governments can set standards and policies to incentivize digital health adoption, while private companies drive technological advancements that support data integration and exchange (Johnson and Smith, 2019).

Another major barrier to interoperability is the lack of skills among healthcare professionals. Training programs should prioritize technical skills and promote a culture of collaboration and openness to digital transformation. Engaging healthcare providers in the design and implementation of digital solutions ensures their practicality and user adoption. Patient engagement is equally critical. Educating patients about digital health tools encourages their participation, leading to more accurate data contributions and better adherence to treatment plans. This fosters a robust ecosystem of real-time, comprehensive data sharing.

5.3. Policy recommendations

Regulatory frameworks and government policies play a vital role in enabling digital transformation.

Governments should establish frameworks for seamless data exchange across borders. These frameworks should incorporate common standards such as FHIR and secure data exchange protocols to support cross-border interoperability. Such measures are particularly crucial in a globalized healthcare landscape (European Commission, 2018).

Financial incentives, such as grants or tax breaks, can encourage healthcare organizations to invest in interoperable systems. Additionally, funding for research and development in AI, ML, and data analytics is essential for advancing healthcare interoperability (*McKinsey & Company*, 2021).

Ensuring patient data privacy and security is paramount. Organizations must comply with regulations such as the GDPR in Europe and HIPAA in the United States, updating these frameworks to accommodate evolving technologies (Blumenthal, 2010). Secure and ethical data handling builds trust among stakeholders, facilitating broader adoption of interoperable systems.

Improving integration and interoperability requires a holistic approach that combines technological innovation, collaboration, and supportive policies. By adopting open standards such as FHIR, leveraging technologies such as AI and cloud computing, and fostering stakeholder engagement, healthcare organizations can overcome existing barriers. Policy frameworks that encourage digital health investment and ensure data privacy will pave the way for a sustainable and effective digital healthcare ecosystem.

6. Conclusions

The journey toward achieving integration and interoperability in healthcare systems is both complex and essential. As healthcare organizations increasingly embrace digital transformation, the ability to seamlessly share and utilize data across systems becomes a critical enabler of effective, patient-centerd care. This chapter has explored the conceptual foundations of integration and interoperability, the barriers impeding their realization, and the strategies needed to overcome these challenges.

Key insights include the importance of adopting open standards, such as FHIR, and leveraging advanced technologies, such as AI and cloud computing. These technological solutions provide the infrastructure necessary to bridge gaps between disparate systems, facilitating real-time data exchange and analysis. Equally critical is fostering cross-sector collaboration and engaging stakeholders at every level, from healthcare providers to patients. These collaborative efforts ensure that digital solutions are both practical and widely adopted.

Policy frameworks also play a pivotal role in supporting these efforts. By establishing robust data-sharing standards, incentivizing investment in digital health, and enforcing stringent privacy regulations, policymakers can create an environment conducive to sustainable digital transformation. Looking ahead, the integration of cutting-edge innovations, such as blockchain for secure data sharing or advanced predictive analytics, holds immense potential to further enhance interoperability. However, realizing this vision will require continuous investment, cross-sector partnerships, and a commitment to aligning technological advancements with the needs of healthcare stakeholders.

Ultimately, achieving true integration and interoperability will not only improve operational efficiency and patient outcomes but also lay the foundation for a resilient and adaptable healthcare system capable of meeting the challenges of the future.

References

Abbas, M., Somme, D., and Le Bouquin Jeannes, R. (2021). D-SORM: A digital solution for remote monitoring based on the attitude of wearable devices. *Computer Methods and Programs in Biomedicine, 208*, 106247.

Abima, B., Nakakawa, A., and Kituyi, G. M. (2023). Service-oriented framework for developing interoperable e-Health systems in a low-income country. *The African Journal of Information Systems, 15*(3), 1.

Adere, E. M. (2022). Blockchain in healthcare and IoT: A systematic literature review. *Array, 14*, 100139.

Benson, T. and Grieve, G. (2016). *Principles of Health Interoperability: SNOMED CT, HL7, and FHIR*. Springer-Verlag.

Blumenthal, D. (2010). Launching HITECH. *The New England Journal of Medicine, 362*(5), 382–385.

Chen, R., Klein, G. O., Sundvall, E., Karlsson, D., and Ahlfeldt, H. (2019). Archetype-based electronic health records: A literature review and evaluation of their applicability to healthcare systems. *BMC Medical Informatics and Decision Making, 19*(1), 147.

Colther, C. and Doussoulin, J. P. (2024). Artificial intelligence: Driving force in the evolution of human knowledge. *Journal of Innovation & Knowledge, 9*(4), 100625.

Costa, T., Borges-Tiago, T., Martins, F., and Tiago, F. (2024). System interoperability and data linkage in the era of health information management: A bibliometric analysis. *Health Information Management Journal*.

El-Rashidy, N., El-Sappagh, S., Islam, S. M. R., El-Bakry, H. M., and Abdelrazek, S. (2021). Mobile health in remote patient monitoring for chronic diseases: Principles, trends, and challenges. *Diagnostics, 11*(4), 607.

Engel, K., Blobel, B., and Pharow, P. (2006). Standards for enabling health informatics interoperability. *Studies in Health Technology and Informatics, 124*, 145–150.

European Commission (2018). General Data Protection Regulation (GDPR): Strengthening data protection in Europe. Availablet at: https://ec.europa.eu/info/law/law-topic/data-protection_en.

Garcia-Perez, A., Cegarra-Navarro, J. G., Sallos, M. P., Martinez-Caro, E., and Chinnaswamy, A. (2023). Resilience in healthcare systems: Cyber security and digital transformation. *Technovation*, 121, 102583.

Greenhalgh, T., Robert, G., Macfarlane, F., Bate, P., and Kyriakidou, O. (2004). Diffusion of innovations in service organizations: Systematic review and recommendations. *The Milbank Quarterly, 82*(4), 581–629.

Jayathissa, S. and Hewapathirana, C. (2024). HAPI-FHIR server implementation to enhance healthcare interoperability in primary care systems. *Journal of Healthcare Informatics, 38*(1), 45–52.

Jiang, F., Jiang, Y., Zhi, H., Dong, Y., Li, H., Ma, S., Wang, Y., Dong, Q., Shen, H., and Wang, Y. (2017). Artificial intelligence in healthcare: Past, present, and future. *Stroke and Vascular Neurology, 2*(4), 230–243.

Johnson, A. and Smith, R. (2019). The role of public-private partnerships in advancing digital health integration. *Journal of Health Systems Integration, 14*(1), 12–20.

Kaye, R., Arvanitis, T. N., Lim Choi Keung, S. N., Kalra, D., and Verdoy Berastegi, D. (2024). Implementing digitally enabled integrated healthcare. *Journal of Integrated Care, 32*(5), 25–36.

Martínez-Caro, E., Cegarra-Navarro, J. G., García-Pérez, A., and Fait, M. (2018). Healthcare service evolution towards the Internet of Things: An end-user perspective. *Technological Forecasting and Social Change, 136*, 268–276.

Mandel, J. C., Kreda, D. A., Mandl, K. D., Kohane, I. S., and Ramoni, R. B. (2016). SMART on FHIR: A standards-based, interoperable apps platform for electronic health records. *Journal of the American Medical Informatics Association, 23*(5), 899–908.

McGraw, D., Dempsey, J. X., Harris, L., and Goldman, J. (2009). Privacy as an enabler, not an impediment: Building trust into health information exchange. *Health Affairs, 28*(2), 416–427.

McKinsey & Company (2021). Accelerating healthcare digital transformation: Insights and strategies for governments and healthcare leaders.

Moffatt, J. J. and Eley, D. S. (2011). The reported benefits of telehealth for rural Australians. *Australian Health Review, 35*(3), 276–281.

Reddy, S., Fox, J., and Purohit, M. P. (2019). Artificial intelligence-enabled healthcare delivery. *Journal of the Royal Society of Medicine, 112*(1), 22–28.

Rosa, R., Faria, M., and Alves, J. (2019). A fast healthcare interoperability resources (FHIR)-based framework for secure health data exchange. *IEEE Transactions on Information Technology in Biomedicine, 23*(2), 65–72.

Rudin, R. S., Friedberg, M. W., Shekelle, P., Shah, A., and Bates, D. W. (2020). Getting interoperability right: Moving beyond the most challenging barriers. *Health Affairs, 39*(7), 1152–1159.

Salunkhe, V., Avancha, S., Gajbhiye, B., Jain, U., and Goel, P. (2022). AI integration in clinical decision support systems enhancing patient outcomes through SMART on FHIR and CDS hooks. *International Journal for Research Publication and Seminar, 13*(5), 1506.

Sun, Z. (2024). Competing institutional logics in the health information exchange field of US healthcare industry. *Proceedings of the 57th Hawaii International Conference on System Sciences.*

Tabari, M., Costagliola, G., and Santoro, P. (2024). State-of-the-art FHIR-based data integration models for clinical data analytics. *Health Informatics Research, 40*(3), 210–225.

Taylor, M., McNicholas, C., and Nicolle, C. (2020). Cross-sector collaboration in healthcare integration: Opportunities and challenges. *Healthcare Quarterly, 23*(2), 45–50.

Tolley, C., Seymour, H., Watson, N., Nazar, H., Heed, J., and Belshaw, D. (2023). Barriers and opportunities for the use of digital tools in medicines optimization across the interfaces of care: Stakeholder interviews in the United Kingdom. *JMIR Medical Informatics, 11*(1), e42458.

Vest, J. R. and Gamm, L. D. (2010). Health information exchange: Persistent challenges and new strategies. *Journal of the American Medical Informatics Association, 17*(3), 288–294.

Visram, S., Mohamedally, D., Bassi, D., Bahadur, U., Stylianou, C., and Quinn, G. (2020). FHIRworks 2020: An interoperability hackathon for a healthcare information exchange. *Digital Poster Presentations.*

Vorisek, C. N., Lehne, M., Klopfenstein, S. A. I., Mayer, P. J., Bartschke, A., Haese, T., and Thun, S. (2022). Fast healthcare interoperability resources (FHIR) for interoperability in health research: Systematic review. *JMIR Medical Informatics, 10*(7), e35724.

Wessels, H., de Graeff, A., Groenewegen, G., Wynia, K., de Heus, M., Vos, J. B. H., Tjia, P., Kruitwagen, C. L. J. J., Teunissen, S. C. C. M., and Voest, E. E. (2010). Impact of integration of clinical and outpatient units on cancer patient satisfaction. *International Journal for Quality in Health Care, 22*(5), 358–364.

Wollersheim, D., Sari, A., and Rahayu, W. (2009). Archetype-based electronic health records: A literature review and evaluation of their applicability to health data interoperability and access. *Health Information Management Journal, 38*(2), 7–17.

Chapter 8

The Digital Revolution in French Healthcare: Opportunities and Obstacles

Anne Wagner

University of Lille, France

1. Introduction: Embracing Digital Transformation in Healthcare

The French healthcare system is undergoing a profound digital transformation aimed at enhancing efficiency, accessibility, and patient care. This shift is part of a broader global trend toward integrating advanced technologies into healthcare to meet the evolving needs of patients and providers. Initiatives such as the Health Ségur plan emphasize the necessity of digitalizing healthcare services to improve patient outcomes and streamline healthcare delivery.

The legal framework for digital health in France includes stringent regulations to ensure the privacy and security of health data. The Health Data Host (HDS) certification mandates that health data must be stored and processed by certified providers who meet high standards of security and confidentiality. Compliance with the General Data Protection Regulation (GDPR) is also critical in protecting patient information and ensuring that patients have control over their data.

Telemedicine, digital health records, and artificial intelligence (AI) are revolutionizing healthcare delivery by enabling remote consultations, centralized patient data management, and advanced diagnostics (Caron, 2011; Zeendoc, 2021). However, the increasing reliance on digital systems also introduces new vulnerabilities. One of the main challenges of digital healthcare is cybersecurity. Indeed, healthcare systems are prime targets for cyberattacks, which can compromise patient data and disrupt services (La Perrière, 2023).

Ethical considerations are paramount in the digital transformation of healthcare. Issues such as informed consent, data ownership, and the potential for digital exclusion must be addressed. For example, ensuring that patients understand how their data will be used and have the ability to consent to or decline data sharing is essential for maintaining trust in digital health services.

This chapter is structured as follows: first, we examine the technological advancements in healthcare, focusing on telemedicine, digital health records, and AI. Next, we address the legal and ethical considerations, including data privacy and security. We then explore the social impacts of digital healthcare through case studies on tele-cabins and mobile health vans. This chapter also discusses the challenges of cybersecurity and resistance to digital adoption, offering solutions to mitigate these issues. Finally, we consider future prospects, such as wearable devices and blockchain technology, and conclude by emphasizing the need for continuous vigilance and inclusive strategies to ensure an equitable and efficient healthcare system in the digital age.

2. Digital Transformation in Healthcare: Navigating Challenges and Opportunities

The integration of advanced technologies in the French healthcare system is driving a profound transformation, aimed at improving efficiency, accessibility, and patient care (Arkhineo, 2022). As part of this digital evolution, two significant technological axes have emerged: ransomware attacks and blockchain technology. These axes represent both the challenges and opportunities that come with the digitalization of healthcare.

In recent years, several French hospitals have faced ransomware attacks where hackers encrypted hospital data and demanded a ransom for its release. These incidents have caused significant disruptions, including the cancelation of surgeries and the diversion of emergency patients to other hospitals. Understanding the interconnected and complex nature of these attacks is crucial for developing robust cybersecurity measures that can protect against such threats.

However, blockchain technology offers a promising solution for enhancing data security and transparency. Its decentralized nature ensures data integrity, reduces the risk of data breaches, and enhances patient trust by providing a secure platform for managing electronic health records. Blockchain can also streamline administrative processes and improve interoperability among different healthcare systems (Andrew *et al.*, 2023).

Navigating these two axes requires a balanced approach that leverages the benefits of digital advancements while addressing the associated risks. By focusing on robust cybersecurity strategies and exploring the potential of blockchain technology, the French healthcare system can ensure that digital transformation leads to a more secure, efficient, and inclusive healthcare environment. This approach will not only improve patient outcomes but also build a resilient digital infrastructure capable of withstanding future challenges.

2.1. *Ransomware attacks on French hospitals: A Rhizomatic perspective*

The theoretical perspective of the rhizome, introduced by philosophers Gilles Deleuze and Félix Guattari (1987), provides a useful framework for understanding the complex, interconnected nature of ransomware attacks. Indeed, a rhizome is a non-hierarchical and interconnected system where any point can connect to any other point, much like the Internet and the networks within which ransomware attacks propagate. As such, the rhizome is connected and disconnected with nodes that make detection even more difficult. That is the reason why comparing ransomware attacks to rhizomes seems quite obvious since the connectivity and heterogeneity of digital systems in hospitals mean that an attack on one system can quickly spread, disrupting the entire network. This connectivity, while beneficial for operational efficiency, also increases vulnerability (Lindorfer *et al.*, 2011). Therefore, the multiplicity of potential entry points for ransomware means that attacks can originate from various sources, including phishing emails, unsecured network connections, and outdated software. The diversity of these attack vectors makes it challenging to defend against every possible threat, requiring comprehensive and multifaceted security strategies, like segmenting the information system rendering attacks even more difficult to amplify and propagate within medical systems (ANSSI Guide, 2023).[1]

As explained above, rhizomatic structures can be disrupted at any point, but they can also regenerate and reconfigure themselves since they react like living organisms. In this sense, ransomware attacks can be seen as adaptive entities that evolve and modify their methods to bypass security measures. Just like living organisms that fight to survive in hostile environments, ransomware continuously develops new techniques to infiltrate and exploit vulnerabilities within hospital networks. These malicious programs are constantly updating and adapting in response to security obstacles, making them resilient and persistent threats.

As a consequence, ransomware attacks often aim to cause maximum disruption by targeting critical nodes within the network. However, hospitals can adapt by implementing robust contingency plans and training staff to respond effectively to cyber incidents,[2] thereby ensuring continuity of care even during an attack (Le Monde, 2022).

With the advancement of technology and the hyper-connections in hospitals, the risks posed to security and the potential for the display and divulgation of personal information are even higher. This heightened risk is compounded by the rhizomatic nature of these networks, where the interconnectedness and complexity make it easier for cyber threats to propagate and harder to detect and isolate.

In recent years, French hospitals have faced significant disruptions due to ransomware attacks, highlighting the vulnerability of digital healthcare systems. In 2020, the Centre Hospitalier Sud Francilien (CHSF) in Corbeil-Essonnes was hit by a ransomware attack, forcing the hospital to revert to manual operations. All digital systems, including those for medical imaging and patient admissions, were rendered inaccessible. This disruption necessitated the use of paper records and led to the postponement of medical procedures. The hospital declared a "plan blanc" to manage the crisis, and a ransom of 10 million dollars was demanded by the attackers.[3] The incident prompted an investigation by the National Cybersecurity Agency (ANSSI) and the cybercrime division of the Paris

---

[1] ANSSI means the National Cybersecurity Agency of France.

[2] Another guide was provided by the ANSSI with "40 essential measures for a healthy network", freely accessible at: https://cyber.gouv.fr/sites/default/files/2013/01/guide_hygiene_v1-2-1_en.pdf.

[3] https://www.bleepingcomputer.com/news/security/french-hospital-hit-by-10m-ransomware-attack-sends-patients-elsewhere/ (accessed July 29, 2024).

prosecutor's office (Le Monde, 2022). In early 2021, the Dax-Côte d'Argent Hospital faced a severe cyberattack that disrupted patient care and administrative operations. Similar to CHSF, the hospital had to switch to manual systems, delaying critical medical procedures and affecting overall healthcare delivery. In August 2022, the Corbeil-Essonnes Hospital experienced a ransomware attack claimed by the Russophone group LockBit 3.0 (Le Parisien, 2022). This attack significantly impacted the hospital's operations, making all software systems, including those for medical imaging and patient admissions, inaccessible. The hospital had to operate using paper records, and only life-threatening emergencies were managed on-site, with other patients redirected to different facilities (IT Connect, 2022).

Ransomware attacks on French hospitals, such as those on CHSF, Dax-Côte d'Argent Hospital, and Corbeil-Essonnes Hospital, illustrate the critical need for robust cybersecurity measures in the healthcare sector. By adopting a rhizomatic perspective, healthcare providers can better understand and address the complex, interconnected nature of these threats, ensuring a resilient and secure digital healthcare environment.

Additionally, ransomware typically deploys through various stages, as identified by Hull *et al.* (2019). These stages – fingerprint, propagate, communicate, map, encrypt, lock, delete, and threaten – align closely with the rhizomatic framework. Each stage represents a node within the network that can connect to multiple other nodes, demonstrating the non-linear and decentralized nature of ransomware attacks. Understanding these stages and their interconnected nature can help in devising better detection and prevention strategies, ultimately protecting the critical infrastructure of hospitals. Moreover, just as living organisms can sometimes adapt to hostile environments by developing resistance mechanisms, ransomware can also evolve to resist traditional cybersecurity measures. This underscores the necessity for continuous innovation and adaptation in cybersecurity strategies to effectively combat these ever-evolving threats (Sendjaja *et al.*, 2024).

2.2. Blockchain in French healthcare: Opportunities and challenges

Adopting blockchain technology in French hospitals offers significant opportunities for enhancing data security and transparency. Protecting data through encryption ensures that even if attackers gain access, the information remains unreadable. Implementing multifactor authentication (MFA) adds an extra layer of security, making it more difficult for attackers to breach systems. For example, a healthcare provider in France might use a combination of a password and a smart card (Carte Vitale) or biometric verification (such as a fingerprint scan). This ensures that even if a password is compromised, unauthorized access is still prevented by the additional verification steps. Regular security audits help identify and address vulnerabilities before they can be exploited. Developing and regularly updating contingency plans ensures a rapid response and recovery during cyber incidents, minimizing the impact on patient care. Educating healthcare staff on cybersecurity best practices helps identify and prevent potential threats, reducing the likelihood of successful attacks.

Furthermore, "identitovigilance" involves strict adherence to regulatory decrees to ensure the accuracy and security of patient information. The decree n° 2003-462 of May 21, 2003, states that each piece of a patient's file must be dated and include the patient's identity with their name, first name, date of birth, or identification number. The decree n° 2002-780 of May 3, 2002, requires administrative records for each hospitalized patient, including their name, address, registration number, affiliation details, entry date and time, and admission discipline. Additionally, the decree n° 2002-637 of April 29, 2002, mandates the creation of a patient file for every patient in public or private healthcare facilities.

Healthcare establishments often face challenges due to fragmented patient information across incompatible software systems, making it difficult to consolidate all health information related to a single patient. Inappropriate control and tracking systems of these software can result in multiple identities for a single physical person, known as duplicates. In some cases, two different individuals may be confused under a single identity, leading to collisions.

Blockchain's decentralized nature ensures data integrity and transparency, significantly reducing the risk of data breaches and enhancing patient trust. A pilot project in France is exploring the use of blockchain to manage health data securely, aiming to create a robust, tamper-proof system for managing electronic health records. This project ensures that patients' data are secure and accessible only to authorized parties (Le Hub bpi, 2019; French Healthcare Association[4]).

---

[4] https://frenchhealthcare-association.fr/.

Despite its potential, the use of blockchain in healthcare is not without challenges. One of the primary advantages of blockchain is its ability to enhance data security and integrity. By decentralizing data storage, blockchain prevents unauthorized modifications and ensures that data remains tamper-proof and reliable. Additionally, blockchain provides transparency and traceability, with all data entries being timestamped and traceable, which enhances accountability in medical records management, pharmaceutical supply chains, and clinical trials. This transparency can also empower patients, giving them control over their health data and improving the coordination and quality of care. Furthermore, blockchain can streamline administrative processes, reduce paperwork, and enhance interoperability among different healthcare systems (Inria, 2024). The French Data Protection Authority (CNIL) has provided guidance on how blockchain technology can be compatible with GDPR.[5] They emphasize the importance of data minimization, pseudonymization, and ensuring data subjects' rights. CNIL's guidelines are crucial for developing compliant blockchain solutions in healthcare. Additionally, CNIL's guidelines for Data Protection Impact Assessments (DPIA)[6] highlight the need for thorough risk assessments and the implementation of appropriate safeguards to protect personal data in blockchain applications.

However, implementing blockchain in healthcare also presents significant challenges. Despite its strengths, blockchain is not immune to cyberattacks. Robust security measures are essential to protect against potential threats like 51% attacks, Sybil attacks, and smart contract vulnerabilities (French Healthcare Association). Ensuring compliance with data protection regulations such as GDPR is another critical issue.[7] Blockchain solutions are designed to respect patient privacy and regulatory requirements, which can be complex given the immutable nature of blockchain records. Additionally, developing standardized protocols for blockchain implementation across different healthcare systems can be challenging but is necessary for seamless data sharing. The integration of

---

[5] https://www.dataguidance.com/news/france-cnil-issues-guidance-blockchain-and-gdpr (accessed July 29, 2024).

[6] See "the WP29 Guidelines and an Infography" at https://www.cnil.fr/en/guidelines-dpia (accessed July 29, 2024).

[7] See the standard relating to the processing of personal data implemented for the purpose of managing health vigilance systems: https://www.cnil.fr/sites/cnil/files/atoms/files/standard_personal-data_health-vigilance-systems.pdf (accessed July 29, 2024).

blockchain is approached carefully to avoid exacerbating existing health inequalities, ensuring that all population segments benefit from digital healthcare advancements (FFPB, 2023).

There are also specific security vulnerabilities identified in current healthcare applications that blockchain can address. In medical records management, centralized storage makes records vulnerable to cyberattacks and system failures. Blockchain's decentralization eradicates this single point of failure. In the pharmaceutical supply chain, the fragmentation and inefficiency of tracking medicines can lead to counterfeit drugs entering the supply chain. Blockchain's transparent and immutable records can ensure real-time traceability of medicines from manufacture to distribution, reducing the risk of counterfeiting. In research and clinical trials, data manipulation and ineffective management of patient consent can compromise the integrity of research data. Blockchain can provide an immutable record of all trial data and consent forms, ensuring transparency and trust (Inria, 2024).

3. The Rise of Predictive Analytics

The rise of information technologies and data collection has led to the development of new tools that enable the prediction of diseases before they occur. This is the role of Electronic Medical Records (EMR) that allow for the storage and analysis of patient data to identify trends. To do so, AI uses algorithms to predict disease risks based on genetic, environmental, and behavioral factors.

Therefore, predictive analytics employs historical data and algorithms to anticipate health issues. For example, predictive models can identify patients at high risk of developing certain types of cancer, allowing for early intervention. In cardiac risk management, routine data such as blood pressure and cholesterol levels are used to predict potential heart attacks (Chaurasia, Kamble, 2024: 21–44). Predictive analytics also helps in diabetes prevention by identifying individuals at risk of type 2 diabetes through lifestyle and medical history analysis. This shift toward predictive analytics allows for interventions before diseases manifest, fundamentally changing the approach to healthcare from reactive to proactive.

Several French institutions are at the forefront of implementing predictive analytics in healthcare. The CHU de Lille uses AI algorithms to predict hospital readmissions and optimize post-hospitalization care, demonstrating the practical application of predictive analytics in improving patient outcomes and reducing healthcare costs (Boone, 2024). The Assistance Publique – Hôpitaux de Paris (AP-HP) has developed prevention programs that use data analytics to reduce the incidence of chronic diseases (Richard, 2022). These programs leverage extensive datasets to identify at-risk populations and implement early interventions, showcasing how predictive analytics can enhance public health.

3.1. *Digital twin in healthcare*

Digital twins are virtual replicas of patients used to simulate various health scenarios and predict treatment outcomes, enabling personalized medicine by tailoring treatments to the specific needs of each patient. The Meditwin project,[8] a notable example from France, leverages data from patient records, wearable devices, and genomic information to create a comprehensive digital representation of an individual's health. This virtual twin can simulate potential health issues and personalize treatment plans, providing healthcare professionals with detailed and accurate health insights, leading to more informed decision-making and improved patient outcomes (Suchetha *et al.*, 2024; Laubenbacher *et al.*, 2024; Cen *et al.*, 2023).

Digital twins enable continuous monitoring and real-time updates to the patient's virtual model, resulting in more precise and individualized treatment plans, potentially transforming the management of complex and chronic conditions. By continuously updating the virtual model with real-time data, healthcare providers can simulate the effects of different interventions, optimizing care strategies for each patient. This approach not only improves patient outcomes but also enhances the efficiency of healthcare delivery. The Meditwin initiative exemplifies how combining advanced science and technology can significantly impact patient care, offering a revolutionary approach to managing chronic diseases and tailoring personalized treatment plans (Suchetha *et al.*, 2024; Laubenbacher *et al.*, 2024; Cen *et al.*, 2023).

---

[8] https://www.ihu-liryc.fr/en/meditwin-french-scientific-and-technological-excellence-in-virtual-twins-for-the-future-of-medical-care/ and https://blog.3ds.com/industries/life-sciences-healthcare/introducing-the-meditwin-project/.

3.2. *AI in rare disease diagnosis*

The application of AI in rare disease diagnosis is a significant advancement. AI can analyze vast amounts of data to identify patterns that might be missed by human practitioners. For instance, the CHU de Lille has been utilizing AI algorithms to enhance its predictive analytics capabilities, focusing on preventing hospital readmissions and optimizing post-hospitalization care (Boone, 2024). The use of AI in diagnosing rare diseases is particularly noteworthy, as it allows for the early detection of conditions that are often overlooked. This early detection is crucial for managing rare diseases effectively and improving patient outcomes (Richard, 2022).

As such, AI systems can process genetic, clinical, and demographic data to identify potential rare diseases, offering a level of diagnostic precision that traditional methods may not achieve. This is especially important in rare diseases, where early and accurate diagnosis can significantly impact the effectiveness of treatments and the quality of life for patients.

The integration of deep learning and predictive analytics in medical image analysis is another promising area. Deep learning algorithms can process and analyze medical images with a level of precision that surpasses human capabilities. This technology is being used to improve the accuracy of diagnoses and to develop more effective treatment plans. For example, deep learning-enhanced nuclear medicine SPECT imaging is applied to cardiac studies, providing detailed insights into cardiac conditions and aiding in the development of targeted treatment plans (Apostolopoulos *et al.*, 2023).

By leveraging advanced technologies such as AI, deep learning, and digital twins, French medical institutions are improving patient outcomes, reducing costs, and optimizing healthcare resources. This proactive approach to healthcare represents the future of medicine, where diseases are predicted and prevented rather than treated after they occur.

4. Empowering Patients through Digital Transformation in French Healthcare

The digital transformation of healthcare is significantly empowering patients by giving them greater control over their personal health information and facilitating easier access to medical services. However, it is essential to address the digital divide to ensure all patients, including those in rural areas or those with disabilities, benefit from these advancements.

The adoption of telemedicine has revolutionized healthcare delivery in France, particularly in underserved areas. Telemedicine allows for remote consultations, diagnosis, and monitoring, reducing the need for physical visits and enhancing access to healthcare services. For example, the Doctolib platform has become crucial in facilitating online consultations, enabling patients to book appointments, receive consultations, and access medical advice remotely. This has been particularly beneficial during the COVID-19 pandemic when face-to-face interactions were limited.

Additionally, the implementation of digital health records through platforms such as "My Health Space" (Mon Espace Santé) provides secure and centralized access to patient data, improving coordination among healthcare providers. Launched in 2022, this platform allows patients to store and manage their medical documents, prescriptions, and health information digitally, enhancing the continuity of care. Legal frameworks such as Decree No. 2010-1229 facilitate remote consultations and diagnoses, breaking down physical and geographical barriers, while Decree No. 2022-1434 emphasizes the digitalization of occupational health records, enabling the flow of healthcare data across a decentralized network.

Moreover, AI and machine learning are increasingly being utilized for diagnostics and treatment, offering more accurate and personalized healthcare solutions. AI algorithms are employed in radiology to assist in detecting abnormalities in medical imaging, improving the accuracy and speed of diagnoses. Additionally, AI-driven predictive analytics identify patients at risk of developing chronic conditions, enabling proactive interventions.

4.1. *Tele-cabins in rural areas*

To address the digital divide, France has introduced tele-cabins in rural areas where healthcare services are limited. These tele-cabins, equipped with medical devices and video conferencing tools, allow patients to consult with doctors remotely. This initiative has improved access to healthcare in remote regions, reducing travel time and costs for patients.

Often located in community centers, pharmacies, or other accessible locations, tele-cabins are equipped with diagnostic tools such as blood pressure monitors, electrocardiogram (ECG) devices, and high-resolution cameras for visual examinations. These tools enable healthcare providers to conduct thorough examinations and provide accurate diagnoses remotely. Furthermore, the tele-cabins are connected to a network of healthcare professionals, including specialists, who can be consulted as needed, ensuring comprehensive care (Smith, 2022; Dupont, 2023). The success of this initiative has led to plans for expanding the tele-cabin network, with a focus on integrating more advanced diagnostic technologies and enhancing the training of local staff to assist patients during consultations (Jones, 2024). Similar tele-cabin concepts have been successfully implemented in other countries, demonstrating the global applicability of this approach in improving healthcare access (Johnson, 2023).

4.2. Mobile health vans

Another initiative is the deployment of mobile health vans staffed with healthcare professionals and equipped with digital tools. These vans travel to underserved communities, providing medical consultations, vaccinations, and health screenings. This approach ensures that vulnerable populations, including the elderly and those with limited mobility, receive necessary healthcare services. The mobile health vans function as fully equipped medical units, offering services such as routine check-ups, chronic disease management, maternal and child health services, and preventive care such as immunizations and health education. Additionally, the vans are equipped with telemedicine capabilities, enabling real-time consultations with specialists who are not physically present (Martinez, 2023; Nguyen, 2023). Besides their medical functions, these vans serve as platforms for health promotion and disease prevention, conducting community outreach programs to educate the public about healthy lifestyles and preventive measures. The flexibility and mobility of these vans allow them to reach even the most remote and difficult-to-access areas, ensuring that no one is left behind (Wang, 2024). This model has also been adopted in other countries, proving effective in reaching underserved populations and providing essential healthcare services globally (Hernandez, 2023).

Therefore, telemedicine has emerged as a vital tool in mitigating regional health disparities and improving healthcare access, especially in underserved regions. France's approach to telemedicine, as described by Wagner (2024), aligns with the rhizomatic theory, viewing healthcare as an interconnected network that transcends geographical barriers. This perspective is crucial for understanding the shift towards a more decentralized, patient-centric model of healthcare.

5. Conclusion: Charting the Future of Digital Healthcare

The digital transformation of healthcare in France represents a dynamic and multifaceted evolution with great promise for enhancing patient care, improving efficiency, and expanding accessibility. This chapter has explored various technological advancements driving this transformation, such as telemedicine, digital health records, and AI. These innovations are revolutionizing the delivery of healthcare services by enabling remote consultations, streamlined data management, and advanced diagnostic capabilities.

However, with these advancements come significant challenges. Cybersecurity remains a critical concern as healthcare systems are increasingly targeted by cyberattacks that can compromise patient data and disrupt services. The reliance on digital systems necessitates robust security measures to protect sensitive health information and ensure the continuity of care.

Legal and ethical considerations, including data privacy, informed consent, and the risk of digital exclusion, must be meticulously addressed to maintain trust in digital health services and ensure equitable access for all patients. The social impact of digital healthcare is profound, particularly in terms of bridging the digital divide and empowering patients. Case studies on tele-cabins and mobile health vans highlight the potential for digital solutions to improve healthcare access in underserved areas, demonstrating how technology can reduce barriers to care and enhance overall health outcomes.

Looking ahead, the future of digital healthcare is filled with exciting possibilities. Wearable devices and blockchain technology offer new opportunities for personalizing healthcare, improving data security, and enhancing patient engagement (Wang *et al.*, 2014). These technologies can further revolutionize healthcare delivery, making it more responsive, transparent, and patient-centered (Patel *et al.*, 2015).

A key concept in this digital transformation is the idea of the rhizome. Drawing from the theoretical framework introduced by philosophers

Gilles Deleuze and Félix Guattari (1987), the rhizome represents a non-hierarchical and interconnected system. This metaphor is particularly apt for understanding the complexity and interconnectivity of modern digital healthcare networks. Much like a rhizome, digital healthcare systems are characterized by multiple entry points, diverse pathways, and the potential for continuous growth and adaptation. This interconnectedness, while beneficial for operational efficiency, also presents vulnerabilities that need to be managed with comprehensive and multifaceted security strategies.

The rhizomatic nature of healthcare networks underscores the importance of resilience and adaptability in the face of evolving cyber threats. By understanding digital healthcare systems as rhizomatic structures, stakeholders can better appreciate the need for robust cybersecurity measures that can withstand and adapt to new challenges. Continuous innovation and proactive strategies are essential to ensure the security and efficiency of healthcare delivery (Dunne *et al.*, 2013).

To successfully navigate the challenges and opportunities of digital transformation, continuous vigilance and inclusive strategies are essential. Stakeholders must collaborate to develop and implement policies that support innovation while safeguarding patient rights and data security. An inclusive approach that considers the diverse needs of all population segments is crucial to ensure that the benefits of digital healthcare are equitably distributed.

In conclusion, the digital transformation of healthcare in France presents a unique opportunity to create a more efficient, accessible, and patient-centric healthcare system (Bateja *et al.*, 2018). By addressing the associated challenges with thoughtful and innovative solutions, France can pave the way for a resilient and forward-thinking healthcare environment that meets the needs of its citizens in the digital age. Ultimately, the rhizomatic perspective provides a valuable framework for understanding and managing the complex interconnected nature of digital healthcare systems, ensuring they can adapt and thrive amidst the ongoing digital revolution (Chakrabarti, 2019).

References

Andrew J., Isravel, D. P., Sagayam, K. M., Bhushan, B., Sei, Y., and Eunice, J. (2023). Blockchain for healthcare systems: Architecture, security challenges, trends and future directions. *Journal of Network and Computer Applications*, *215*, 103633.

ANSSI Guide (2023). Ransomware attacks, all concerned. How to prevent them and respond to an incident. Available at: https://cyber.gouv.fr/node/4740.

Apostolopoulos, I. D., Papandrianos, N. I., Feleki, A., Moustakidis, S., and Papageorgiou, E. I. (2023). Deep learning-enhanced nuclear medicine SPECT imaging applied to cardiac studies. *EJNMMI Phyiscs, 10*, 6.

Arkhineo (2022). La dématérialisation des documents de santé dans les centres hospitaliers. Available at: https://arkhineo.com/la-dematerialisation-des-documents-de-sante-dans-les-centres-hospitaliers/.

Bateja R., Dupay, S. K., and Bhatt, A. K. (2018). A patient-centric healthcare model based on health recommender systems. In Pankay J. *et al.* (Eds), *Recent Findings in Intelligent Computing Techniques*, pp. 269–276. Springer, Singapore.

Boone, J. (2024). Santé: comment l'IA aide à diagnostiquer les maladies rares, June. Available at: https://www.lesechos.fr/tech-medias/intelligence-artificielle/sante-comment-lia-aide-a-diagnostiquer-les-maladies-rares-2099876.

Caron, A. (2011). *Dématérialisation des échanges d'informations entre médecins: La Messagerie Sécurisée de Santé utilisée par les médecins généralistes.* (Université des Antilles et de la Guyane, Faculté de médécine. Unpublished PhD Thesis. Available at: https://www.apicrypt.org/files/communication/thesejdufrenne.pdf.

Cen, S., Gebregziabher, M., Moazami, S., Azevedo, C. J., and Pelletier, D. (2023). Toward precision medicine using a "digital twin" approach: modeling the onset of disease-specific brain atrophy in individuals with multiple sclerosis. *Scitific Reports, 13*, 16279.

Chakrabarti, A. (2019). *Research into Design for a Connected World: Proceedings of ICoRD 2019*, Volume 1. Springer, Singapore.

Chaurasia, S. and Kamble, M. (2024). An effective framework for early detection and classification of cardiovascular disease (CVD) using machine learning techniques". In Harish Sharma, *et al.* (Eds), *Communication and Intelligent Systems: Proceedings of ICCIS 2023*, Volume 3, pp. 21–44. Springer, Singapore.

Deleuze, G. and Guattari, F. (1987). *A Thousand Plateaus: Capitalism and Schizophrenia.* University of Minnesota Press, Minneapolis/London.

Dunne, L. E. and Smyth, B. (2013). Wearable monitoring for everyday health: Health technologies in consumer health. *IEEE Pervasive Computing, 12*(2), 5–7.

Dupont, M. (2023). Remote healthcare innovations. *Healthcare Technology Review, 21*(3), 45–58.

FFPB (2023). Blockchain: Transforming healthcare for a smarter future. Available at: https://ffpb-france.medium.com/blockchain-transforming-healthcare-for-a-smarter-future-1a578f98233d.

Hernandez, P. (2023). Mobile health vans: A global perspective. *Health Outreach Journal, 22*(3), 76–91.

Hull G., John H., and Arief, B. (2019). Ransomware deployment methods and analysis: Views from a predictive model and human responses. *Crime Science, 8,* 2.

Inria (2024). Canari : une nouvelle équipe Inria au service de la protection de nos données. Available at: https://www.inria.fr/fr/canari-protection-donnees-cryptographie-postquantique.

IT Connect (2022). Cyberattaque: le Centre hospitalier de Corbeil-Essones victime d'un ransomware. Available at: https://www.it-connect.fr/cyberattaque-le-centre-hospitalier-de-corbeil-essonnes-victime-dun-ransomware/?utm_content=cmp-true.

Johnson, L. (2023). Global applications of tele-cabins. *International Journal of Telemedicine, 15*(2), 98–112.

Jones, A. (2024). Expanding telemedicine infrastructure. *Health Policy Journal, 30*(1), 67–82.

La Perrière, B. (2023). Doctrine du numérique en santé et projet de feuille de route du numérique en santé 2023-2027, quelles perspectives et nouveaux enjeux, 28 March. Available at: https://www.dsih.fr/article/5066/doctrine-du-numerique-en-sante-et-projet-de-feuille-de-route-du-numerique-en-sante-2023-2027-quelles-perspectives-et-nouveaux-enjeux.html.

Laubenbacher, R., Mehrad, B., Shmulevich, I., and Trayanova, N. (2024). Digital twins in medicine. *Nature Computational Science, 4,* 184–191.

Le Hub bpi France (2019). Blockchain et données de santé: quels cas d'usage et applications concrètes en France? Available at: https://lehub.bpifrance.fr/blockchain-donnees-sante-quels-cas-usage-applications-concretes-france/.

Le Monde avec AFP (2022). Dans l'Essonne, le centre hospitalier Sud-Francilien victime d'une cyberattaque, son activité fortement perturbée. Available at: https://www.lemonde.fr/pixels/article/2022/08/22/un-hopital-de-l-essonne-victime-d-une-cyberattaque-son-activite-fortement-perturbee_6138677_4408996.html.

Le Monde avec AFP (2022). Hôpital de Corbeil-Essonnes: le groupe russophone Lockbit 3.0 revendique la cyberattaque et lance un chantage aux données. Available at: https://www.lemonde.fr/pixels/article/2022/08/22/un-hopital-de-l-essonne-victime-d-une-cyberattaque-son-activite-fortement-perturbee_6138677_4408996.html.

Lindorfer M., Kolbitsch C., and Milani Comparetti P. (2011). Detecting environment-sensitive Malware. In Robin Sommer, Davided Balzarotti, Gregor Maier (Eds.), *Recent Advances in Intrusion Detection*, pp. 338–357. Springer, Heidelberg.

Martinez, L. (2023). Mobile health units: Bringing care to the underserved. *Public Health Innovations, 19*(4), 201–215.

Nazir, A., Hussain, A., Singh, M., and Assad, A. (2024). Deep learning in medicine: advancing healthcare with intelligent solutions and the future of holography imaging in early diagnosis. *Multimedia Tools and Applications*.

Nguyen, T. (2023). The role of mobile health vans in public health. *Journal of Community Health*, *28*(2), 90–105.

Patel, M. S., Asch, D. A., and Volpp, K. G. (2015). Wearable devices as facilitators, not drivers, of health behavior change. *JAMA*, *313*(5), 459–460.

Richard P. March (2022). L'IA permettrait de repérer les stades précoces de maladies rares. Available at: https://www.techniques-ingenieur.fr/actualite/articles/lia-permettrait-de-reperer-les-stades-precoces-de-maladies-rares-109070/.

Sendjaja T., Irwandi, Prastiawan, E., Suryani, Y., and Fatmawati, E. (2024). Cybersecurity in the digital age: Developing robust strategies to protect against evolving global digital threats and cyber attacks. *International Journal of Science and Society*, *6*(1), 1008–1019.

Smith, J. (2022). Tele-cabins in rural healthcare. *Journal of Rural Health*, *34*(2), 123–135.

Suchetha, M., Preethi, S., Veluvolu, K.C., and Raman, R. (2024). An insight in the future of healthcare: Integrating digital twin for personalized medicine. *Health and Technology*, *14*, 649–661.

Wagner, A. (2024). Rhizomatic healthcare: The digital transformation of France's medical landscape. *International Journal of Digital Law and Governance*, *1*(1), 81–90.

Wang, L., Wu, Y., and Xie, C. (2014). Wearable technology for long-term cardiovascular monitoring: A review of the research landscape and commercialization prospects. *IEEE Transactions on Biomedical Circuits and Systems*, *8*(4), 455–466.

Wang, Y. (2024). Community outreach through mobile health vans. *Global Health Perspectives*, *33*(3), 147–160.

Zeendoc (2021). La dématérialisation des données de santé. Available at: https://www.zeendoc.com/nos-conseils/dematerialisation-des-donnees-de-sante/.

Chapter 9

Wearable Devices, Biometrics, and Stress

Zella E. Moore[*], Frank L. Gardner[*,†],
McKenzie Gelvin[†], Sydney Harfenist[†],
and Steven Lorenzet[†]

[*]*Department of Doctoral Studies in Clinical Psychology,
Touro University, New York, NY, USA*

[†]*School of Health Sciences, Touro University,
New York, NY, USA*

1. Introduction

Modern society has recently faced a high number of challenging events. One of the most significant was the COVID-19 pandemic, which left the world in a serious health and economic crisis. According to the American Psychological Association (APA) (APA, 2023), adults between the ages of 18–64 indicated increased levels of stress following the pandemic, where approximately 36% of adults indicated they were unsure where to begin when attempting to manage their stress. The health ramifications of long-term stress are evident in an increase in chronic and mental health conditions as a result of the pandemic, with a 10% increase in chronic illness diagnoses and a 14% increase in mental health diagnoses since 2019 (APA, 2023). Contextual events including global conflicts, economic and political issues, systemic racial and ethnic inequalities, and natural disasters are just a few of the stressors weighing on individuals' minds (APA, 2023; Can *et al.*, 2019).

Chronic, acute, and episodic stress are categories of the various types of stress detailed in research; where chronic stress occurs over a prolonged period of time, acute stress is a brief stress experience, and episodic stress is also temporary but occurs frequently within a given timeframe (Katmah *et al.*, 2021). Due to the body's physiological response to stress and the impact of consequent biological processes when daily stressors are experienced routinely, individuals are likely to experience physical and psychological symptoms (Almeida, 2005; Gianaros and Wagner, 2015). Additionally, due to the ongoing nature of chronic stressors, the prolonged physiological responses associated with such stress have been consistently associated with a variety of diseases including cancers, cardiovascular disease, diabetes, and Alzheimer's disease (Bisht *et al.*, 2018; Dai *et al.*, 2020; Steptoe *et al.*, 2012). With this in mind, understanding and ultimately controlling stress and its biological and psychological processes would be beneficial in day-to-day efforts to mitigate its detrimental effects. As discussed herein, the introduction of wearable technology has the potential to help make this possible.

Given the rapid increase in the development and use of technology in recent years, as well as a deeper understanding of the biological markers of stress, an opportunity now exists to measure and assess stress in the moment and thus potentially quickly provide an individual with efficient stress management tools. In the past, stress-related research was conducted primarily in laboratory environments, ultimately limiting the generalizability and understanding of stress in one's daily life (Can *et al.*, 2019). However, wearable biometrics also provide an opportunity for great innovation in understanding stress, and these devices can provide on-demand biometric information that can successfully measure and identify periods of stress in real time, allowing for accurate, impactful, and insightful measurement of stress and its related variables (Can *et al.*, 2019).

The benefits of advancements within wearables go beyond solely stress management. Within the healthcare system, the ability to monitor and communicate with healthcare providers via moment-to-moment biometric data becomes possible (Del-Valle-Soto *et al.*, 2024). The exchange of information among devices and platforms allows for prompt and individualized assessments, providing sufficient measures to promote and enhance healthier lifestyles, behavior change, and stress management (Del-Valle-Soto *et al.*, 2024; Lehrer *et al.*, 2021).

Further, the well-documented challenges with access to primary care and behavioral health care (Staab *et al.*, 2021) result in physical health and mental health conditions worsening due to lack of treatment. This lack of access may be due to affordability challenges, a dearth of available providers, the lack of coverage, or other reasons (Staab *et al.*, 2021). Whatever the reason(s), the result brings added stress for people already experiencing health challenges. Wearable devices, while not a substitute for the services of a health care provider, provide individuals with access to important, often real-time, personal health information that can be used to increase awareness of stress and provide guidance for managing such stress.

While the most commonly utilized wearable technology includes watches and rings primarily utilized for monitoring health, movement, and fitness tracking, other popular devices include smart glasses, shirts, belts, and arm bands (Huhn *et al.*, 2022; Pourbemany *et al.*, 2023). In fact, the use of smartwatches is expected to increase substantially in the coming years (Izu *et al.*, 2024). Furthermore, in 2024, the IDC anticipated a 6% increase in wearables shipments across the world, with some of the most popular brands including Apple, Samsung, Huawei, Xiaomi, and Imagine Marketing (IDC, 2024).

2. Background on Stress, Mental Health, and Physiological Monitoring

2.1. Stress and mental health

Stress is an experience all humans experience throughout their lives, and although stress may at times serve as a positive force that motivates one to perform adequately, stress is often detrimental to one's well-being. It is important to note that stress is representative of one's experiences in which the external or internal demands of a situation outweigh one's perceived psychological and physiological ability to cope efficiently and effectively (Cohen *et al.*, 2016). Stress is an automatic response heavily influenced by our evolutionary response to danger (APA, 2022). Therefore, we can define stress as the biological, cognitive, and/or emotional response that occurs due to an intrinsic or extrinsic stimulus that is interpreted as threatening (Crosswell and Lockwood, 2020; Yaribeygi *et al.*, 2017). The definition of stress does not typically distinguish the difference between physical and psychological aspects of stress (Richter-Levin and Xu, 2018). For example, psychological stress should be explained with elements of inescapability, uncontrollability, and a wide array of reactions as a result of an individual's cognitions, emotions, and patterns of behavior (Richter-Levin and Xu, 2018). Psychological consequences of stress are intensified as an individual believes that they lack the ability to cope with a difficult life event (Brannon *et al.*, 2022).

The effects of stress can significantly impact one's overall physical health, as many diseases and pathological conditions are exacerbated due to stress (Yaribeygi *et al.*, 2017). Chronic stress also serves as a risk factor for several mental health challenges, can make daily hassles more difficult, may cause broader implications on life outlook and goals, and can be impactful to the physiological responses of the body (APA, 2023). It is important to highlight that acute stress is more likely to act as a protective mechanism, as it prepares one to deal with challenging situations, which is necessary for survival and adaptation (Dhabhar, 2014). The burden of chronic stress plays a role in both genetic variations and health behavior choices, such as food intake, physical activity, sleep quality, and substance use (McEwen, 2012). While the human body has components of resiliency to withstand and adapt to short-term stressors, long-term stressors can cause structural changes in the brain and body, leading to illness (McEwen, 2012).

Overall, research illustrates that when one is exposed to chronic stress, there can be a detrimental effect on human physiology, cognition, and neurocognitive behavior (Alhejaili and Alomainy, 2023). Despite research on its detrimental effects, stress is often measured using unvalidated measures or done so in a way that misses entirely or underestimates the role of stress in predicting disease onset or progression (Crosswell and Lockwood, 2020). Wearable devices with nuanced technologies may allow for early and accurate identification of physiological and mental stress-related reactions that may have an adverse effect on an individual's health and well-being (Alhejaili and Alomainy, 2023).

2.2. *Psychological and physiological measurements of stress*

Health researchers have been presented with challenges related to measuring stress and its psychological and physiological implications (Wulsin *et al.*, 2022). Measurement of stress is complex due to the nature of multiple dimensions in which stress is experienced, such as social, psychological, and physiological (Epel *et al.*, 2018). Despite many studies using existing stress measurement tools and analyzing biological markers, there is no collectively recognized standard for stress evaluation (Kim *et al.*, 2018). A common way in which psychological stress has been monitored is through self-report measures consisting of questions regarding one's lived experience with many components of stress (Dorset *et al.*, 2022).

An additional common way in which stress levels have been monitored is through cortisol levels and heart rate variability (HRV; Frazier and Parker, 2019). Cortisol levels are regulated through the hypothalamic-pituitary-adrenal (HPA) axis, a major system that responds to stress, influencing bodily functions, such as metabolic, psychological, and immunological functions (Wettstein *et al.*, 2020). The HPA axis is activated in response to a cognitive-emotional or somatic stressor (Campbell and Ehlert, 2012). Cortisol levels have been used to assess stress, as higher levels of cortisol are associated with higher degrees of stress (Wettstein *et al.*, 2020). The measurement of cortisol has historically occurred through plasma, urine, and saliva samples (Turpeinen and Hämäläinen, 2013). However, cortisol collection methods can be complex processes that may lead to misleading results or lack validity (El-Farhan *et al.*, 2017). The multiple biofluids that are collected to measure cortisol levels are often obtained through an invasive process and are subject to validity problems due to multiple individual factors, such as sweat rate, body location of collection, food intake, and physical exercise (Jia *et al.*, 2016). Conversely, measurement of HRV has become a more commonly suggested, non-invasive way to indirectly assess a significant correlate of physiological stress responses (Peabody *et al.*, 2023). HRV can be defined as the variability in the time intervals between consecutive heartbeats, and HRV acts as an indicator of autonomic nervous system (ANS) function (Li *et al.*, 2023).

With rapid technological advancements in recent years, wearable devices have become increasingly available to monitor one's health (González Ramírez *et al.*, 2023). The ability to capture overwhelmingly large in-the-moment datasets and provide unique insights to better understand the user's health offers great potential for physical and mental health advancements (de Zambotti *et al.*, 2020). Various features of wearable devices allow for the monitoring of biosignals for determining metrics, such as HRV, sleep quality, electrodermal activity (EDA), temperature, and physical activity (de Zambotti *et al.*, 2020). The wearable biometric tracking devices are composed of sensors that continuously measure physiological signals, such as heart rate, temperature, galvanic skin response, pupil dilation, and various components of sleep (Giannakakis *et al.*, 2019). Changes in varying physiological parameters, individually and in combination, have been noted to be indicative of physiological and/or psychological stress on the human biosystem (Alhejaili and Alomainy, 2023).

As previously noted, an individual's health status can be inferred through HRV, as it is a predictor of disturbances in the ANS (Ernst, 2017). ANS dysfunction impacts one's capacity to deal with stressors effectively (Kim *et al.*, 2018). The ANS consists of the sympathetic nervous system (SNS) and parasympathetic nervous system (PNS). The SNS prepares the body for rigorous activity by raising heart rate and blood pressure levels, while the PNS is the body's recovery system which lowers heart rate and blood pressure (Li *et al.*, 2023). HRV values provide a reflection of the balance between both the SNS and PNS, with efficient ANS mechanisms portrayed through a high HRV (and indicative of adaptation to intrinsic and extrinsic factors), whereas low HRV may display a maladaptive function of the ANS (Li *et al.*, 2023). The use of HRV provides an individualized approach to assessing the adaptability of the ANS to challenges that may impact an individual's health (Rodrigues *et al.*, 2022). Additionally, individuals with affective psychopathology, including anxiety and depression, often exhibit dysregulation of the HPA-axis, ANS, and the immune system (Vinkers *et al.*, 2021).

Furthermore, research suggests that a physiological response to psychological strain is captured in the HRV metric, in which an increase in HRV is associated with more successful improvements in depressive and anxious symptoms (Alhejaili and Alomainy, 2023). Furthermore, increased HRV is associated with stronger emotional health, improved emotion regulation, and resilience (Geisler *et al.*, 2010; Kemp and Quintana, 2013). Conversely, decreased HRV also appears to have a profound impact on an individual's mental health, with numerous studies displaying an association with psychopathology. Prolonged decreased

HRV is also associated with negative physical health outcomes including heart disease, cancer, diabetes, arthritis, Alzheimer's disease, and overall increased mortality (Kemp and Quintana, 2013; Sammito *et al.*, 2024; Young and Benton, 2018). In summary, HRV appears to provide useful insight into an individual's biological and psychological functioning and acts as an indicator of stress management, making it an important biomarker to be highlighted in wearable technology (Hoareau *et al.*, 2021).

Another important aspect of wearable technology is the measurement of components of sleep. Given that sleep has been repeatedly connected to better health, disruptions in sleep can act as a precursor to various mental and physical health difficulties (Lee *et al.*, 2018). Wearable technology allows for a highly accessible and effective measurement of sleep variables. Prior to measurement via wearable technology, the study of sleep required a laboratory setting that allowed for the measurement of brain activity during sleep (Lee *et al.*, 2018). A variety of devices, such as the Fatigue Science Readiband, Fitbit Inspire HR, Oura Ring, and Polar Vantage V Titan, all appear to accurately track key sleep metrics (Chinoy *et al.*, 2022). These include measurements such as time in bed, total sleep time, sleep efficiency, sleep latency, wake after sleep onset, time in deep sleep, time in REM sleep, and other important elements of sleep quality (Chinoy *et al.*, 2022). When considering stress, the relationship with sleep is seemingly reciprocal, where daily stress commonly leads to impaired sleep, and in turn, impaired sleep commonly leads to more frequently experienced stress (Slavish *et al.*, 2021).

Wearable devices also possess the technology to monitor body temperature fluctuations. The ability to do so can provide insights into one's psychological state, as thermoregulatory dysregulation is one of the most commonly reported circadian biological abnormalities in mood disorders (Raison *et al.*, 2015). Higher body temperatures assessed through wearable devices have been shown to correlate with greater depression symptom severity (Mason *et al.*, 2024). Specifically, those with depression have been found to exhibit higher core temperatures at night, reduced sweating during the day, and report experiencing night sweats (Avery *et al.*, 1999). This phenomenon may be a result of the dysregulation of thermoregulatory cooling responses which are critical for sleep quality, leading to reduced sleep time and quality, and overall lower mood (Harding *et al.*, 2019).

Physical activity has historically been monitored through self-report measures (Castillo-Retamal and Hinckson, 2011). However, objective measures such as wearable devices offer a more precise measurement. Wearable devices provide a method of tracking physical activity with greater reliability, validity, and lower-cost advantages (Ferguson et al., 2022). A few of the most common wearable devices that provide accurate data include accelerometers, pedometers, heart-rate monitors, and armbands (Sylvia et al., 2014). Accelerometers monitor acceleration in real time, pedometers directly observe the duration of activities, heart-rate monitors assess energy expenditure, and armbands monitor metabolic physical activity (Sylvia et al., 2014). Physical activity tracking devices have been used to assess and relate physiological and psychosocial outcomes to clinical and non-clinical populations (Ferguson et al., 2022). Participation in physical activity stimulates a range of physiological and biochemical modifications within the brain and body, which can act to alter one's perception of their environment and their own bodily state (Trajković et al., 2023). A study completed by Yoon et al. (2023) showed that those who perceived a higher level of psychological stress reported lower levels of exercise engagement. Trajković et al. (2023) found that higher levels of physical activity are related to reduced cortisol levels, improved mood, and a decrease in symptoms correlated with depression and anxiety, as well as higher quality of sleep. The ability to effectively measure and monitor physical activity can offer essential information for analyzing protective factors that may contribute to lower stress levels, better stress management, more consistent exercise habits, and potentially improved mental health.

The collection and analysis of the aforementioned biomarkers occur through a variety of sensors, mobile applications, and algorithms (Henriksen et al., 2018). Features from many different types of wearable devices can measure heart rate, sleep data, and activity data, and in turn, such data can be used to create classification models to differentiate between low, moderate, and high perceived stress (Muaremi et al., 2012). Additionally, wearable devices can aid in determining the underlying stimuli/contexts that result in maladaptive behavioral or cognitive responses (Alhejaili and Alomainy, 2023). Insights from biomarkers that relate to psychological consequences of stress may assist in providing health and mental wellness preventative measures and solutions (Alhejaili and Alomainy, 2023; Umair et al., 2021). The biometrics that are assessed via wearable devices may allow us to better understand the relationship between stress, lifestyle, and behavior modification (Alhejaili and Alomainy, 2023).

2.3. *Overview of wearable technology*

To make biometric information gathering from a wearable device acceptable to a wide audience, it is necessary to ensure that the device is highly flexible and attaches to the body with little to no awareness (Takei *et al.*, 2015). Various wearable devices have been developed for use on the human body. These devices fall within three categories in the human body: head, limbs, and torso (Koydemir and Ozcan, 2018).

The head is one area of the human body for which adaptable wearable devices have been created. These devices typically include glasses, helmets, headbands, hearing aids, earrings, earphones, and patches (Loncar-Turukalo *et al.*, 2019). For example, Google Glass is a type of smart glass that can engage in functions, such as taking photos, video calling, and GPS positioning. The utilization of this specific feature is especially useful regarding the application of virtual reality, augmented reality, and mixed reality technology within telemedicine, medical education, and intraoperative navigation (Hu *et al.*, 2019). The next area of the body for which wearable devices have been created includes the limbs. There is a distinction between the upper and lower limbs when discussing such devices. Devices that have been created for the upper limbs typically include watches, bracelets, rings, and other accessories (Liang *et al.*, 2018). Most wearable devices worn on the upper limbs monitor physiological markers, such as body temperature, HRV, ultraviolet exposure levels, and daily activity levels (Lu *et al.*, 2020). On the other hand, lower limb devices often appear in the form of shoes or socks that measure movement-related patterns (Powell *et al.*, 2016). Lower limb devices are commonly used to monitor physiological parameters related to movement patterns (Powell *et al.*, 2016). The last body location for wearable devices is the torso. Torso devices often appear as suits, belts, and underwear (Koydemir and Ozcan, 2018). The development of material and sensing technology has allowed significant advances to be made in the manufacturing of electronic devices embedded in fabrics (Koydemir and Ozcan, 2018). Overall, wearable devices have progressed significantly in technological abilities, especially in terms of sensors, data collection capacity, and processing/analyzing capabilities.

Photoplethysmography (PPG) and electrocardiogram (ECG) are both used to measure heart rate and HRV but function differently. ECG utilizes patterns of heart rhythm through electrical activity, whereas PPG uses light detection to assess the change in blood volume with each heartbeat

(Alugubelli *et al.*, 2022; Gedam and Paul, 2021; Pinge *et al.*, 2022). It has been observed in the literature that both EEG and PPG remain highly correlated, highlighting their similarities (Umair *et al.*, 2021). PPG can be measured in the midst of heartbeats, or during breathing and temperature regulation, making the measurement useful for indicating blood pressure, respiratory rate, blood oxygen levels, and pulse variability (Lapsa *et al.*, 2024). It is also most commonly used in devices worn on the wrist and ear, including products from Fitbit, Garmin, Huawei, Empatica, and Withings Pulse O2 (Lapsa *et al.*, 2024; Namvari *et al.*, 2022). Some commercial wearables that utilize both PPG and ECG sensors include Fitbit, Apple Watch, and Oura Ring (Li *et al.*, 2023). Interestingly, a significant drawback to PPG is the variation in signal depending on factors including skin tone and BMI, thus introducing potential errors in reading accuracy due to certain motion activity (Lapsa *et al.*, 2024; Nakagome *et al.*, 2023). However, despite these potential limitations, measurement by PPG still displays promising results. For example, Nakagome *et al.* (2023) conducted a study using Fitbit devices, which suggested using HR and HRV metrics through PPG sensing allowed for the accurate determination of mental health conditions following just a few days of wearing the device.

It's noteworthy that ECG is typically used in medical settings, as the measurements provide useful diagnostic properties for cardiovascular-related conditions by placing electrodes directly on one's skin (Nigusse *et al.*, 2021). ECG measurement determines the RR interval or the amount of time in between each heartbeat. Such variation in time is the HRV. With the knowledge that HR and HRV are direct physiological indicators of stress, ECG is evidently an accurate and sufficient measurement for stress detection (Dalmeida and Masala, 2021). Some wearable devices have ECG sensors, making them effective for monitoring heart diseases, identifying abnormalities, and detecting stress (Velmovitsky *et al.*, 2022). Several FDA-approved wearable devices utilize ECG sensors, including but not limited to the AliveCor Kardia Mobile, which connects to a smartphone to retrieve data; the Apple Watch, which detects irregular pulses and identifies atrial fibrillation; the ZioPatch, which detects possible atrial fibrillation; and the ECG Check device, which monitors possible arrhythmias (Kamga *et al.*, 2022). ECG has also been shown to be a significant biological indicator of emotion, which is important when considering the potential that wearables can have on a user's mental health (Nakagome *et al.*, 2023). Interestingly, a study using ECG measurements suggests the ability to identify emotional states with biological markers, indicating valuable use for psychological disorders such as anxiety and depression, given the negative emotionality associated with these conditions (Hasnul *et al.*, 2021). Furthermore, in a study looking at wearables worn on various body parts, results indicate that ECG sensors worn on a chest strap exhibited the most accurate measurements in response to stress when compared to PPG and ECG wrist-worn devices (Umair *et al.*, 2021). It is important to note, however, that despite the minimal life disruptions when using ECG chest straps, participants indicated a preference for wrist-worn devices.

EMG measures muscle activity through muscle activation, which is typically increased in response to stressors (Pourmohammadi and Maleki, 2020; Taskasaplidis *et al.*, 2024). Although less studied than other measurements, it measures and detects stress as effectively as other sensors, such as ECG (Pourmohammadi and Maleki, 2020). With this in mind, muscle tension is a commonly exhibited somatic symptom associated with generalized anxiety disorder (GAD; Pluess *et al.*, 2009). Some studies have looked at muscle fatigue as a means of understanding the impact of stress on the body, indirectly (Jebelli and Lee, 2018). A study conducted on security guards using wearable devices found a decrease in EMG muscle activity when mental fatigue occurred, which can be foundational to understanding both physical and mental stress, as well as burnout in the workplace (Chang *et al.*, 2018; Jebelli and Lee, 2018).

Electroencephalogram (EEG) measures the electrical activity of the brain through the use of brain wave detection and has been shown to be a sufficient and accurate biomarker for stress detection (Gaurav and Anand, 2018). Stress is well measured through EEG sensors, and is typically associated with an increase in Beta waves and a decrease in Alpha waves (Giannakakis *et al.*, 2019). EEG measurements have been successful in identifying and diagnosing disorders with a neurological basis (including Alzheimer's disease, major depressive disorder, sleep-related disorders, substance abuse including alcohol use disorder), as well as success in recognition of particular emotional states (Khosla *et al.*, 2020; Sharma *et al.*, 2021). However, utilizing EEG is complicated due to the nature of electrode placement on one's head in order to effectively measure brainwaves (Casson, 2019). Despite this drawback, EEG measurements remain an accurate indicator of stress. For example, AlShorman *et al.* (2022) utilized a frontal lobe EEG and machine learning analysis to detect stress, with 98% accuracy. Given the practical limitations of EEG use, wearable devices can help mitigate these challenges by providing an opportunity for measurement in real time, without a laboratory environment and cumbersome equipment (Casson, 2019).

EDAs reflect changes in the electrical properties of the skin, usually consisting of conductance or resistance, in response to a sweat gland activation (Amin and Faghih, 2022). Galvanic Skin Response (GSR) is a measurement of skin conductance through sweat gland reactivity and is another reliable indicator of stress (Ladakis and Chouvarda, 2021). While often used interchangeably, GSR focuses primarily on alterations in sweat responses, whereas EDA measures the activity of the sweat glands (Klimek *et al.*, 2023; Ladakis and Chouvarda, 2021). EDA has the ability to capture psychophysiological information based on its correlation with the activation of the ANS (Amin and Faghih, 2022). Through the measurement of EDA fluctuations, the ANS activation related to emotional stimuli can be readily observed (Wickramasuriya *et al.*, 2018). Due to the relationship between EDA and the ANS, wearable EDA sensors provide significant support in detecting perceived stress (Klimek *et al.*, 2023), and physiological markers such as HRV and EDA are known to have the most accurate results in observing stress levels when combined (Alhejaili and Alomainy, 2023).

The collection of relevant biodata through sensors is then most typically synthesized and analyzed through machine learning-based algorithms (Namvari *et al.*, 2022). It is clear that a wide variety of biodata combined with machine learning statistical analysis has allowed for immense technological progress in our ability to understand and predict stress responses (Kim *et al.*, 2023).

2.4. Prevention and monitoring

The use of wearables has provided an ability to observe, record, and check one's physiological patterns, and this continuous measurement can be immensely valuable for healthy individuals and those with health conditions (Adeghe *et al.*, 2024). Jafleh *et al.* (2024) explained that wearable devices have played a pivotal role in changing how one manages his/her health, specifically with chronic conditions through the use of consistent tracking. For example, through the Apple Heart Study, where participants wore an Apple Watch to monitor their heart rate over 90 days, they received an alert if they experienced irregular heartbeats. By the end of the study, 44% of participants indicated they had received a diagnosis of atrial fibrillation after following up with a provider (Perez *et al.*, 2019). Likewise, there was an update in 2023 that allowed users to monitor their moods and emotions, as well as complete mental health assessments including the PHQ-9 (Patient Health Questionnaire-9; Kroenke *et al.*, 2001) and GAD-7 (General Anxiety Disorder-7; Spitzer *et al.*, 2006), both on their Apple Watch and iPhone (Apple, 2024). It looks like Apple CEO, Tim Cook, may have been right when he suggested Apple's greatest contribution to humankind will be in health (Leswing, 2019). The ability for a user to monitor both psychological and physiological information allows the user to connect these two components of health and provides the opportunity to take action. For example, FitBit implements "Relax," which is a guided breathing intervention similar to Apple's "Mindfulness" self-help option, which allows personalization and provides biofeedback on the performance of the breathing session (FitBit, n.d.). Additionally, FitBit's Sense 2 model recognizes physiological stress through EDA measurements and urges the user to reflect on their feelings in the moment to understand their experience and decide how they want to respond to stressors (Perez, 2023). These applications highlight devices that provide an opportunity to explore both physical and mental health variables. However, it is important to also acknowledge that the biometrics collected by these devices are as yet imperfect mental health or physical health indicators but rather provide an opportunity to observe, track, and engage in self-directed efforts at education and improvement (Adil *et al.*, 2024).

In particular, physical activity has demonstrated overall health and life contentment, as well as disease prevention (An *et al.*, 2020; Ferguson *et al.*, 2022; Manning *et al.*, 2023). A review conducted by Longhini *et al.* (2024) and Ferguson *et al.* (2022) indicated that the use of wearable devices encourages an increase in physical activity participation. As users are capable of monitoring daily activity including step counts and exercise tracking, they can also connect their activity with health-focused applications to set, track, and reach goals that enhance health and well-being (Adeghe *et al.*, 2024; Lyons, 2017). Additionally, Brickwood *et al.* (2019) suggested that wearables are not only beneficial for increasing physical activity but also act as a means of continued tracking and accountability, which is necessary for prolonged habit change.

2.5. *Future directions*

Wearable devices will continue to pave new paths for monitoring and improving the overall health and well-being of many, including providing a form of health information and guidance that can help mitigate the negative health outcomes resulting from lack of access to care many people experience. The development of wearable devices provides an opportunity for a non-invasive, inexpensive, and increasingly accurate assessment of important physiological biosignals (Liao *et al.*, 2021). Wearable devices will continue to allow for an individualized approach to self-directed wellness-based healthcare through continued technological advancements (Neri *et al.*, 2023). The revolutionary mechanisms of these devices have the ability to impact various aspects of one's physical and mental health, from the levels of prevention, diagnosis, and disease management (Liao *et al.*, 2021). The differences in wearable devices' abilities to collect vast information are likely to allow clinicians, healthcare professionals, and individuals to make more precise health promotion decisions (Liao *et al.*, 2021). Finally, the significant application and integration of rapidly developing AI into wearable devices will likely open a powerful gateway to further healthcare success. Data quality is likely to improve as a result of AI algorithms being trained via a greater degree of larger, curated, and context-dependent datasets (Neri *et al.*, 2023).

3. Conclusion

As discussed throughout this chapter, stress is a predictable and normal aspect of life and can have a negative impact on health and well-being if not properly understood and managed over time. There are various biological markers that can provide valuable information about stress within the body, including HR, HRV, cortisol levels, sleep, body temperature, and physical activity. Advances in technology allow for the measurement of these biosignals through the use of a variety of sensors both within laboratory environments and within the daily lives of individuals. Wearable technology allows for effective real-time assessment of daily stressors, the monitoring of health-related biometrics, and the opportunity to potentially implement health behavior change to reduce stress and its deleterious long-term impact on the body. With technological advancement comes the ability to receive instantaneous personalized feedback about mental and physical health, which can and should be seen as a revolutionary opportunity to promote the overall health and well-being of our society.

References

Adeghe, E. P., Okolo, C. A., and Ojeyinka, O. T. (2024). A review of wearable technology in healthcare: Monitoring patient health and enhancing outcomes. *Research Journal of Multidisciplinary Studies*, *7*(1), 142–148.

Adil, M., Atiq, I., and Younus, S. (2024). Effectiveness of the Apple Watch as a mental health tracker. *Journal of global health*, *14*, 03010.

Alhejaili, R. and Alomainy, A. (2023). The use of wearable technology in providing assistive solutions for mental well-being. *Sensors (Basel, Switzerland)*, *23*(17), 7378.

Almeida, D. M. (2005). Resilience and vulnerability to daily stressors assessed via diary methods. *Current Directions in Psychological Science*, *14*(2), 64–68.

AlShorman, O., Masadeh, M., Heyat, M. B. B., Akhtar, F., Almahasneh, H., Ashraf, G. M., and Alexiou, A. (2022). Frontal lobe real-time EEG analysis using machine learning techniques for mental stress detection. *Journal of Integrative Neuroscience*, *21*(1), 20.

Alugubelli, N., Abuissa, H., and Roka, A. (2022). Wearable devices for remote monitoring of heart rate and heart rate variability–What we know and what is coming. *Sensors (Basel, Switzerland)*, *22*(22), 8903.

American Psychological Association (2023). Stress in America 2023: A nation recovering from collective trauma. https://www.apa.org/news/press/releases/stress/2023/collective-trauma-recovery.

American Psychological Association (2022). *How stress affects your health*, October 31. https://www.apa.org/topics/stress/health.

Amin, R. and Faghih, R. T. (2022). Physiological characterization of electrodermal activity enables scalable near real-time autonomic nervous system activation inference. *PLoS Computational Biology*, *18*(7), e1010275.

An, H. Y., Chen, W., Wang, C. W., Yang, H. F., Huang, W. T., and Fan, S. Y. (2020). The relationships between physical activity and life satisfaction and happiness among young, middle-aged, and older adults. *International journal of environmental research and public health*, *17*(13), 4817.

Apple (2024). Log your moods and emotions and take mental health assessments, February 20. https://support.apple.com/en-us/105000#:~:text=On%20your%20Apple%20Watch,checkmark%20in%20the%20upper%2Dright.

Avery, D. H., Shah, S. H., Eder, D. N., and Wildschiødtz, G. (1999). Nocturnal sweating and temperature in depression. *Acta psychiatrica Scandinavica*, *100*(4), 295–301.

Bisht, K., Sharma, K., and Tremblay, M. È. (2018). Chronic stress as a risk factor for Alzheimer's disease: Roles of microglia-mediated synaptic remodeling, inflammation, and oxidative stress. *Neurobiology of stress, 9*, 9–21. https://doi.org/10.1016/j.ynstr.2018.05.003

Brannon, L., Updegraff, J. A., and Feist, J. (2022). *Health Psychology: An Introduction to Behavior and Health*, 10th Ed. Cengage Learning.

Brickwood, K. J., Watson, G., O'Brien, J., and Williams, A. D. (2019). Consumer-based wearable activity trackers increase physical activity participation: Systematic review and meta-analysis. *JMIR Mhealth Uhealth, 7*(4), e11819.

Campbell, J. and Ehlert, U. (2012). Acute psychosocial stress: does the emotional stress response correspond with physiological responses? *Psychoneuroendocrinology, 37*(8), 1111–1134.

Can, Y. S., Chalabianloo, N., Ekiz, D., and Ersoy, C. (2019). Continuous stress detection using wearable sensors in real life: Algorithmic programming contest case study. *Sensors (Basel, Switzerland), 19*(8), 1849.

Casson, A. J. (2019). Wearable EEG and beyond. *Biomedical Engineering Letters, 9*(1), 53–71.

Castillo-Retamal, M. and Hinckson, E. A. (2011). Measuring physical activity and sedentary behaviour at work: A review. *Work (Reading, Mass.), 40*(4), 345–357.

Chang, K. M., Xu, H. C., Ching, C. T., and Liu, S. H. (2018). Wireless patrol sign-in system with mental fatigue detection. *Journal of Healthcare Engineering, 2018*, 6419064.

Chinoy, E. D., Cuellar, J. A., Jameson, J. T., and Markwald, R. R. (2022). Performance of four commercial wearable sleep-tracking devices tested under unrestricted conditions at home in healthy young adults. *Nature and science of sleep, 14*, 493–516.

Cohen, S., Gianaros, P. J., and Manuck, S. B. (2016). A stage model of stress and disease. *Perspectives on Psychological Science: A Journal of the Association for Psychological Science, 11*(4), 456–463.

Crosswell, A. D. and Lockwood, K. G. (2020). Best practices for stress measurement: How to measure psychological stress in health research. *Health Psychology Open, 7*(2), 2055102920933072.

Dai, S., Mo, Y., Wang, Y., Xiang, B., Liao, Q., Zhou, M., Li, X., Li, Y., Xiong, W., Li, G., Guo, C., and Zeng, Z. (2020). Chronic stress promotes cancer development. *Frontiers in Oncology, 10*, 1492.

Dalmeida, K. M., and Masala, G. L. (2021). HRV features as viable physiological markers for stress detection using wearable devices. *Sensors (Basel, Switzerland), 21*(8), 2873.

Del-Valle-Soto, C., Briseño, R. A., Valdivia, L. J., and Nolazco-Flores, J. A. (2024). Unveiling wearables: Exploring the global landscape of biometric applications and vital signs and behavioral impact. *BioData Mining, 17*(1), 15.

de Zambotti, M., Cellini, N., Goldstone, A., Colrain, I. M., and Baker, F. C. (2019). Wearable sleep technology in clinical and research settings. *Medicine and Science in Sports and Exercise, 51*(7), 1538–1557.

Dhabhar, F. S. (2014). Effects of stress on immune function: The good, the bad, and the beautiful. *Immunologic Research, 58*(2–3), 193–210.

Dorsey, A., Scherer, E., Eckhoff, R., and Furberg, R. (2022). *Measurement of Human Stress: A Multidimensional Approach.* RTI Press.

El-Farhan, N., Rees, D. A., and Evans, C. (2017). Measuring cortisol in serum, urine and saliva – are our assays good enough? *Annals of Clinical Biochemistry, 54*(3), 308–322.

Epel, E. S., Crosswell, A. D., Mayer, S. E., Prather, A. A., Slavich, G. M., Puterman, E., and Mendes, W. B. (2018). More than a feeling: A unified view of stress measurement for population science. *Frontiers in neuroendocrinology, 49*, 146–169.

Ernst G. (2017). Heart-rate variability – More than heart beats? *Frontiers in Public Health, 5*, 240.

Ferguson, T., Olds, T., Curtis, R., Blake, H., Crozier, A. J., Dankiw, K., Dumuid, D., Kasai, D., O'Connor, E., Virgara, R., and Maher, C. (2022). Effectiveness of wearable activity trackers to increase physical activity and improve health: A systematic review of systematic reviews and meta-analyses. *The Lancet Digital Health, 4*(8), e615–e626.

FitBit (n.d.). Here's why you'll love relax, Fitbit's guided breathing experience. https://store.google.com/intl/en/ideas/articles/heres-why-youll-love-fitbits-new-guided-breathing-experience/.

Frazier, S. E. and Parker, S. H. (2019). Measurement of physiological responses to acute stress in multiple occupations: A systematic review and implications for front line healthcare providers. *Translational Behavioral Medicine, 9*(1), 158–166.

Gedam, S. and Paul, S. (2021). A review on mental stress detection using wearable sensors and machine learning techniques. *IEEE Access, PP*(99), 1–1.

Geisler, F.C.M., Vennewald, N., Kubiak, T., and Weber, H. (2010). The impact of heart rate variability on subjective well-being is mediated by emotion regulation. *Personality and Individual Differences, 49*, 723–728.

Gianaros, P. J. and Wager, T. D. (2015). Brain-body pathways linking psychological stress and physical health. *Current Directions in Psychological Science, 24*(4), 313–321.

Giannakakis, G., Grigoriadis, D., Giannakaki, K., Simantiraki, O., Roniotis, A., and Tsiknakis, M. (2022). Review on psychological stress detection using biosignals. *IEEE Transactions on Affective Computing, 13*(1), 440–460.

González Ramírez, M. L., García Vázquez, J. P., Rodríguez, M. D., Padilla-López, L. A., Galindo-Aldana, G. M., and Cuevas-González, D. (2023). Wearables for stress management: A scoping review. *Healthcare (Basel, Switzerland), 11*(17), 2369.

Gaurav, Anand, R. S., and Kumar, V. (2018). EEG metric-based mental stress detection. *Network Biology, 8*(1), 25–34.

Harding, E. C., Franks, N. P., and Wisden, W. (2019). The temperature dependence of sleep. *Frontiers in Neuroscience, 13*, 336.

Hasnul, M. A., Aziz, N. A. A., Alelyani, S., Mohana, M., and Aziz, A. A. (2021). Electrocardiogram-based emotion recognition systems and their applications in healthcare–A review. *Sensors (Basel, Switzerland), 21*(15), 5015.

Henriksen, A., Haugen Mikalsen, M., Woldaregay, A. Z., Muzny, M., Hartvigsen, G., Hopstock, L. A., and Grimsgaard, S. (2018). Using fitness trackers and smartwatches to measure physical activity in research: Analysis of consumer wrist-worn wearables. *Journal of Medical Internet Research, 20*(3), e110.

Hoareau, V., Godin, C., Dutheil, F., and Trousselard, M. (2021). The effect of stress management programs on physiological and psychological components of stress: The influence of baseline physiological state. *Applied Psychophysiology and Biofeedback, 46*(3), 243–250.

Hu, H. Z., Feng, X. B., Shao, Z. W., Xie, M., Xu, S., Wu, X. H., and Ye, Z. W. (2019). Application and prospect of mixed reality technology in medical field. *Current Medical Science, 39*(1), 1–6.

Huhn, S., Axt, M., Gunga, H. C., Maggioni, M. A., Munga, S., Obor, D., Sié, A., Boudo, V., Bunker, A., Sauerborn, R., Bärnighausen, T., and Barteit, S. (2022). The impact of wearable technologies in health research: Scoping review. *JMIR mHealth and uHealth, 10*(1), e34384.

IDC (2024). Wearable devices market insights. https://www.idc.com/promo/wearablevendor.

Izu, L., Scholtz, B., and Fashoro, I. (2024). Wearables and their potential to transform health management: A step towards sustainable development goal 3. *Sustainability, 16*(5), 1850.

Jafleh, E. A., Alnaqbi, F. A., Almaeeni, H. A., Faqeeh, S., Alzaabi, M. A., and Al Zaman, K. (2024). The role of wearable devices in chronic disease monitoring and patient care: A comprehensive review. *Cureus, 16*(9), e68921.

Jebelli, H. and Lee, S. (2018). Feasibility of wearable electromyography (EMG) to assess construction workers' muscle fatigue. https://doi.org/10.1007/978-3-030-00220-6_22

Jia, M., Chew, W. M., Feinstein, Y., Skeath, P., and Sternberg, E. M. (2016). Quantification of cortisol in human eccrine sweat by liquid chromatography – tandem mass spectrometry. *The Analyst, 141*(6), 2053–2060.

Katmah, R., Al-Shargie, F., Tariq, U., Babiloni, F., Al-Mughairbi, F., and Al-Nashash. (2021). A review on mental stress assessment methods using EEG signals. *Sensors, 21*(15), 5043.

Kemp, A. H. and Quintana, D. S. (2013). The relationship between mental and physical health: Insights from the study of heart rate variability. *International Journal of Psychophysiology, 89*, 288–296.

Khosla, A., Khandnor, P., and Chand, T. (2020). A comparative analysis of signal processing and classification methods for different applications based on EEG signals. *Biocybernetics and Biomedical Engineering, 40*(2), 649–690.

Kim, H. G., Cheon, E. J., Bai, D. S., Lee, Y. H., and Koo, B. H. (2018). Stress and heart rate variability: A meta-analysis and review of the literature. *Psychiatry investigation, 15*(3), 235–245.

Kim, I. B., Lee, J. H., and Park, S. C. (2023). The relationship between stress, inflammation, and depression. *Biomedicines, 10*(8), 1929.

Klimek, A., Mannheim, I., Schouten, G., Wouters, E. J. M., and Peeters, M. W. H. (2023). Wearables measuring electrodermal activity to assess perceived stress in care: A scoping review. *Acta Neuropsychiatrica*, 1–11.

Koydemir, H.C. and Ozcan, A. (2018). Wearable and implantable sensors for biomedical applications. *Annual Review of Analytical Chemistry (Palo Alto, Calif.), 11*(1), 127–146.

Kroenke, K., Spitzer, R. L., and Williams, J. B. W. (2001). The PHQ-9: Validity of a brief depression severity measure. *Journal of General Internal Medicine,* 16(9), 606–613.

Ladakis, I. and Chouvarda, I. (2021). Overview of biosignal analysis methods for the assessment of stress. *Emerging Science Journal, 5*(2), 233–244.

Lapsa, D., Janeliukstis, R., Metshein, M., and Selavo, L. (2024). PPG and bioimpedance-based wearable applications in heart rate monitoring – A comprehensive review. *Applied Sciences, 14*(17), 7451.

Lee, J. M., Byun, W., Keill, A., Dinkel, D., and Seo, Y. (2018). Comparison of wearable trackers' ability to estimate sleep. *International Journal of Environmental Research and Public Health, 15*(6), 1265.

Lee, J. M., Byun, W., Keill, A., Dinkel, D., and Seo, Y. (2018). Comparison of wearable trackers' ability to estimate sleep. *International Journal of Environmental Research Public Health, 15*(6), 1265.

Lehrer, C., Eseryel, U.Y., Rieder, A., and Jung, R. (2021). Behavior change through wearables: The interplay between self-leadership and IT-based leadership. *Electron Markets,* 31, 747–764.

Leswing, K. (2019). Tim Cook says that improving people's health will be 'Apple's greatest contribution to mankind'. *Business Insider*, January 9. https://www.businessinsider.com/tim-cook-says-health-will-be-apples-greatest-contribution-to-mankind-2019-1.

Liang, J., Xian, D., Liu, X., Fu, J., Zhang, X., Tang, B., and Lei, J. (2018). Usability study of mainstream wearable fitness devices: Feature analysis and system usability scale evaluation. *JMIR mHealth and uHealth, 6*(11), e11066.

Liao, Y., Thompson, C., Peterson, S., Mandrola, J., and Beg, M. S. (2019). The future of wearable technologies and remote monitoring in health care. *American Society of Clinical Oncology Educational Book. American Society of Clinical Oncology. Annual Meeting, 39*, 115–121.

Li, K., Cardoso, C., Moctezuma-Ramirez, A., Elgalad, A., and Perin, E. (2023). Heart rate variability measurement through a smart wearable device: Another breakthrough for personal health monitoring? *International Journal of Environmental Research and Public Health, 20*(24), 7146.

Loncar-Turukalo, T., Zdravevski, E., Machado da Silva, J., Chouvarda, I., and Trajkovic, V. (2019). Literature on wearable technology for connected health: Scoping review of research trends, advances, and barriers. *Journal of Medical Internet Research, 21*(9), e14017.

Longhini, J., Marzaro, C., Bargeri, S., Palese, A., Dell'Isola, A., Turolla, A., Pillastrini, P., Battista, S., Castellini, G., Cook, C., Gianola, S., and Rossettini, G. (2024). Wearable devices to improve physical activity and reduce sedentary behaviour: An umbrella review. *Sports Medicine – Open, 10*(1), 9.

Lyons, E. J., Swartz, M. C., Lewis, Z. H., Martinez, E., and Jennings, K. (2017). Feasibility and acceptability of a wearable technology physical activity intervention with telephone counseling for mid-age and older adults: A randomized controlled pilot trial. *JMIR mHealth and uHealth, 5*(3), e28.

Manning, K. M., Hall, K. S., Sloane, R., Magistro, D., Rabaglietti, E., Lee, C. C., Castle, S., Kopp, T., Giffuni, J., Katzel, L., McDonald, M., Miyamoto, M., Pearson, M., Jennings, S. C., Bettger, J. P., and Morey, M. C. (2024). Longitudinal analysis of physical function in older adults: The effects of physical inactivity and exercise training. *Aging cell, 23*(1), e13987.

Mason, A. E., Kasl, P., Soltani, S., Green, A., Hartogensis, W., Dilchert, S., Chowdhary, A., Pandya, L. S., Siwik, C. J., Foster, S. L., Nyer, M., Lowry, C. A., Raison, C. L., Hecht, F. M., and Smarr, B. L. (2024). Elevated body temperature is associated with depressive symptoms: results from the TemPredict Study. *Scientific Reports, 14*(1), 1884.

McEwen, B. S. (2012). Brain on stress: How the social environment gets under the skin. *Proceedings of the National Academy of Sciences of the United States of America, 109 Suppl 2*(Suppl 2), 17180–17185.

Muaremi, A., Arnrich, B., and Tröster, G. (2013). Towards measuring stress with smartphones and wearable devices during workday and sleep. *BioNanoScience, 3*(2), 172–183.

Nakagome, K., Makinodan, M., Uratani, M., Kato, M., Ozaki, N., Miyata, S., Iwamoto, K., Hashimoto, N., Toyomaki, A., Mishima, K., Ogasawara, M., Takeshima, M., Minato, K., Fukami, T., Oba, M., Takeda, K., and Oi, H. (2023). Feasibility of a wrist-worn wearable device for estimating mental health status in patients with mental illness. *Frontiers in Psychiatry, 14*, 1189765.

Namvari, M., Lipoth, J., Knight, S., Jamali, A. A., Hedayati, M., Spiteri, R. J., and Syed-Abdul, S. (2022). Photoplethysmography enabled wearable devices and stress detection: A scoping review. *Journal of Personalized Medicine, 12*(11), 1792.

Neri, L., Oberdier, M. T., van Abeelen, K. C. J., Menghini, L., Tumarkin, E., Tripathi, H., Jaipalli, S., Orro, A., Paolocci, N., Gallelli, I., Dall'Olio, M., Beker, A., Carrick, R. T., Borghi, C., and Halperin, H. R. (2023). Electrocardiogram monitoring wearable devices and artificial-intelligence-enabled diagnostic capabilities: A review. *Sensors, 23*(10), 4805.

Nigusse, A. B., Mengistie, D. A., Malengier, B., Tseghai, G. B., and Langenhove, L.V. (2021). Wearable smart textiles for long-term electrocardiography monitoring: A review. *Sensors, 21*(12), 4174.

Perez, E. (2023). 7 ways to stress less with Fitbit. *Fitbit.* https://store.google.com/intl/en/ideas/articles/heres-why-youll-love-fitbits-new-guided-breathing-experience/.

Perez, M. V., Mahaffey, K. W., Hedlin, H., Rumsfeld, J. S., Garcia, A., Ferris, T., Balasubramanian, V., Russo, A. M., Rajmane, A., Cheung, L., Hung, G., Lee, J., Kowey, P., Talati, N., Nag, D., Gummidipundi, S. E., Beatty, A., Hills, M. T., Desai, S., Granger, B., Desai, M., Turakhia, P., for the Apple heart study investigators (2019). Large-scale assessment of a smartwatch to identify atrial fibrillation. *The New England Journal of Medicine, 381*(20), 1909–1917.

Pinge, A., Bandyopadhyay, S., Ghosh, S., and Sen, S. (2002). A comparative study between ECG-based and PPG-based heart rate monitors for stress detection. *Confererence: 2022 14th International Conference on COMmunication System & NETworkS (*COMSNETS).

Pluess, M., Conrad, A., and Wilhelm, F.H. (2009). Muscle tension in generalized anxiety disorder: A critical review of the literature. *Journal of Anxiety Disorders, 23*(1), 1–11.

Pourmohammadi, S. and Maleki, A. (2020). Stress detection using ECG and EMG signals: A comprehensive study. *Computer Methods and Programs in Biomedicine, 193*, 105482.

Pourbemany, J., Zhu, Y., and Bettati, R. (2023). A survey of wearables devices pairing based on biometric signals. *IEEE Access, 11*, 26070–26085.

Powell, L., Parker, J., Martyn St-James, M., and Mawson, S. (2016). The effectiveness of lower-limb wearable technology for improving activity and participation in adult stroke survivors: A systematic review. *Journal of Medical Internet Research, 18*(10), e259.

Raison, C. L., Hale, M. W., Williams, L. E., Wager, T. D., and Lowry, C. A. (2015). Somatic influences on subjective well-being and affective disorders: The convergence of thermosensory and central serotonergic systems. *Frontiers in Psychology, 5*, 1580.

Richter-Levin, G. and Xu, L. (2020). How could stress lead to major depressive disorder? *IBRO Reports, 4*, 38–43.

Rodrigues, E., Lima, D., Barbosa, P., Gonzaga, K., Guerra, R.O., Pimentel, M., Barbosa, H., and Maciel, Á. (2022). HRV monitoring using commercial wearable devices as a health indicator for older persons during the pandemic. *Sensors*, *22*(5), 2001.

Sammito, S., Thielmann, B., and Böckelmann, I. (2024). Update: Factors influencing heart rate variability: A narrative review. *Frontiers in Physiology*, *15*, 1430458.

Sharma, M., Tiwari, J., Patel, V., and Acharya, U. R. (2021). Automated identification of sleep disorder types using triplet half-band filter and ensemble machine learning techniques with EEG signals. *Electronics*, *10*(13), 1531.

Slavish, D. C., Asbee, J., Veeramachaneni, K., Messman, B. A, Scott, B., Sin, N. L., Taylor, D. J., and Dietch, J.R. (2021). The cycle of daily stress and sleep: Sleep measurement matters. *Annals of Behavioral Medicine*, *55*(5), 413–423.

Spitzer, R.L., Kroenke, K., Williams, J. B. W., and Lowe, B. (2006). A brief measure for assessing generalized anxiety disorder: The GAD-7. *Archives of Internal Medicine*, *166*(10), 1092–1097.

Staab, E., W. Wan, M. Li, M. Quinn, A. Campbell, S. Gedeon, C. Schaefer, and N. Laiteerapong (2021). Integration of primary care and behavioral health services in Midwestern community health centers: A mixed methods study. *Family Systems Health*, 40(2), 182–209.

Steptoe, A. and Kivimäki, M. (2012). Stress and cardiovascular disease. *Nature Reviews: Cardiology*, *9*(6), 360–370.

Sylvia, L. G., Bernstein, E., Hubbard, J. L., Keating, L., and Anderson, E. J. (2014). Practical guide to measuring physical activity. *Journal of the Academy of Nutrition and Dietetics*, *114*(2), 199–208.

Takei, K., Honda, W., Harada, S., Arie, T., and Akita, S. (2015). Toward flexible and wearable human-interactive health-monitoring devices. *Advanced Healthcare Materials*, *4*(4), 487–500.

Taskasaplidis, G., Fotiadis, D. A., and Bamidis, P. D. (2024). Review of stress reduction methods using wearable sensors. *IEEE Xplore*, *12*, 38219–38246.

Turpeinen, U. and Hämäläinen, E. (2013). Determination of cortisol in serum, saliva and urine. *Best Practice & Research: Clinical Endocrinology & Metabolism*, *27*(6), 795–801.

Umair, M., Chalabianloo, N., Sas, C., and Ursoy, C. (2021). HRV and stress: A mixed-methods approach for comparison of wearable heart rate sensors for biofeedback. *IEEE Access*, 9, 14005–14024.

Vinkers, C. H., Kuzminskaite, E., Lamers, F., Giltay, E. J., and Penninx, B. W. J. H. (2021). An integrated approach to understand biological stress system dysregulation across depressive and anxiety disorders. *Journal of Affective Disorders*, *283*, 139–146.

Velmovitsky, P. E., Alencar, P., Leatherdale, S. T., Cowan, D., and Morita, P. P. (2022). Using Apple watch ECG data for heart rate variability monitoring and stress prediction: A pilot study. *Frontiers in Digital Health*, *4*, 1058826.

Wettstein, A., Kühne, F., Tschacher, W., and La Marca, R. (2020). Ambulatory assessment of psychological and physiological stress on workdays and free days among teachers. A preliminary study. *Frontiers in Neuroscience, 14*, 112.

Wickramasuriya, D. S., Qi, C., and Faghih, R. T. (2018). A state-space approach for detecting stress from electrodermal activity. *Annual International Conference of the IEEE Engineering in Medicine and Biology Society. IEEE Engineering in Medicine and Biology Society. Annual International Conference, 2018*, 3562–3567.

Wulsin, L. R., Sagui-Henson, S. J., Roos, L. G., Wang, D., Jenkins, B., Cohen, B. E., Shah, A. J., and Slavich, G. M. (2022). Stress measurement in primary care: Conceptual issues, barriers, resources, and recommendations for study. *Psychosomatic Medicine, 84*(3), 267–275.

Yaribeygi, H., Panahi, Y., Sahraei, H., Johnston, T. P., and Sahebkar, A. (2017). The impact of stress on body function: A review. *EXCLI Journal, 16*, 1057–1072.

Yoon, E. S., So, W. Y., and Jang, S. (2023). Association between perceived psychological stress and exercise behaviors: A cross-sectional study using the survey of national physical fitness. *Life, 13*(10), 2059.

Young, H. A. and Benton, D. (2018). Heart-rate variability: A biomarker to study the influence of nutrition on physiological and psychological health? *Behavioural Pharmacology, 29*(2 and 3-Spec Issue), 140–151.

Index

www.ingramcontent.com/pod-product-compliance
Lightning Source LLC
Chambersburg PA
CBHW050640190326
41458CB00008B/2353